Pickard's Guide to Minimally Invasive Operative Dentistry

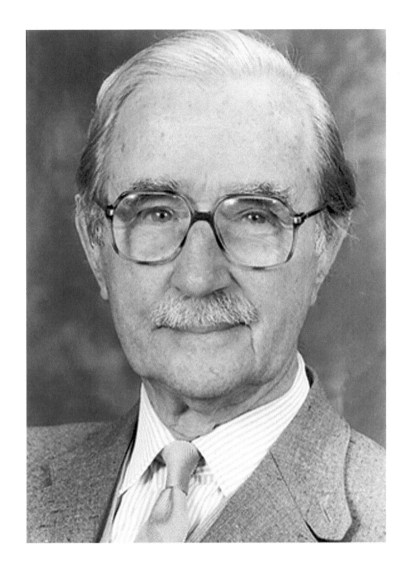

Professor H. M. Pickard 1909–2002

Pickard's Guide to Minimally Invasive Operative Dentistry

TENTH EDITION

Avijit Banerjee

Professor of Cariology and Operative Dentistry
Honorary Consultant/Clinical Lead, Restorative Dentistry
Head of Conservative and MI Dentistry
King's College London Dental Institute at Guy's, King's College
and St Thomas' Hospitals,
King's Health Partners, London, UK
and
Visiting Professor of Restorative Dentistry, Oman Dental
College, Oman

Timothy F. Watson

Professor of Biomaterials and Restorative Dentistry
King's College London Dental Institute at Guy's,
King's College and St Thomas' Hospitals,
King's Health Partners, London, UK

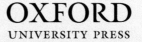

OXFORD
UNIVERSITY PRESS

OXFORD
UNIVERSITY PRESS

Great Clarendon Street, Oxford, OX2 6DP,
United Kingdom

Oxford University Press is a department of the University of Oxford.
It furthers the University's objective of excellence in research, scholarship,
and education by publishing worldwide. Oxford is a registered trade mark of
Oxford University Press in the UK and in certain other countries

Seventh Edition published in 1996
Eighth Edition published in 2003
Ninth Edition published in 2011

Impression: 7

Published in the United States of America by Oxford University Press
198 Madison Avenue, New York, NY 10016, United States of America

British Library Cataloguing in Publication Data
Data available

Library of Congress Control Number: 2014959003

ISBN 978-0-19-871209-1

Printed and bound in Great Britain by Ashford Colour Press Ltd., Gosport, Hampshire.

Foreword

It was a 'great pleasure and honour' to have been asked to prepare the foreword for the previous edition of Pickard. To have been asked to prepare the foreword for the new-look, new-style tenth edition is a huge honour and pleasure, given that I have been selected to introduce this ground-breaking book in the rapidly developing field of patient-centred and oral healthcare team-delivered, biologically based, minimally invasive, minimum intervention (MI) care dentistry. To practise operative dentistry in any other way in the twenty-first century is not only old-fashioned, but contrary to the best interests of patients.

If Professor Pickard were alive today, I believe he would be delighted to be associated with the ways in which operative dentistry and relevant dental biomaterials science have evolved and developed since his pioneering days as a leader in the field, and to see the tenth edition of his book promote and encourage modern MI approaches to the clinical practice of operative dentistry. I also anticipate that Professors Bernard Smith and Edwina Kidd, who were entrusted with the 'Manual' by Pickard, will be most pleased to see this new edition pushing back the frontiers of the clinical practice of operative dentistry. As described in the accompanying preface by the present custodians of the Pickard legacy—Professors Avijit Banerjee and Timothy Watson—the 'Manual' has undergone major change during the preparation of the new, more user-friendly tenth edition, including a change in title to reflect all that is new in the state-of-the-art management of diseased and damaged teeth and tooth tissues. Professors Banerjee and Watson are to be congratulated not just on the excellence and attractiveness of the tenth edition of Pickard, but on their forward-looking approach and leadership in the promotion of patient-centred, minimally invasive, minimum intervention care dentistry.

In my foreword to the ninth edition of Pickard, I referred to a 'watershed between the traditional and modern art and science of operative dentistry.' With the publication of this tenth edition of Pickard, the transition from traditional, mechanistic, and traumatic to modern, truly tooth-preserving, conservative operative dentistry may be considered to have been largely completed, one of the major outstanding challenges being the translation of all that is described and beautifully illustrated in this book into the everyday clinical practice of dentistry. For established practitioners and teachers this may necessitate a fundamental change in thinking and approach. For students (present and future) a door has been opened to an innovative, much more challenging approach to patient-centred care. For future researchers, this book highlights the many different ways in which operative dentistry and relevant dental biomaterials science must continue to evolve.

From the style developed by Professors Banerjee and Watson, it is apparent that they fully appreciate the challenge that this tenth edition of Pickard poses in terms of putting aside traditional thinking and long-established procedures and techniques in order to embrace new, preventatively orientated concepts and principles. Of particular note is the introduction in this new edition of the '5Rs' concept to enhance and extend the life expectancy of restorations, and in turn teeth, through a slowing down of the so-called 'restorative death spiral.' If you are unfamiliar with the '5Rs' concept, that alone is sufficient justification for you to acquire and study this book.

I applaud the work of Banerjee and Watson and unreservedly recommend this new edition of Pickard to all members of the oral healthcare team. I very much hope that the new knowledge and understanding that it imparts will be widely and effectively translated by all team members into clinical practice in the best interests of existing and future generations of patients. For this to happen, it is hoped that teachers will revise their curricula accordingly, and funders of oral healthcare provision will critically review the extent to which their systems allow and encourage the practice of modern, evidence-based, minimally invasive operative dentistry as described in this book.

Professors Banerjee and Watson have produced a state-of-the-art text on operative dentistry. We must now rise to the challenge to practise twenty-first rather than late twentieth-century operative dentistry. Anyone who reads this book will be hard pressed to find good reason for continuing to practise 'old-style' traditional operative dentistry. The move to 'new-style' MI operative dentistry may be challenging, but it will bring countless benefits both to patients and to the profession.

Nairn Wilson CBE DSc (*h.c.*) FDS FFD FFGDP FCDSHK FACD FADM FHEA FKC

Preface to the tenth edition

The first edition of this textbook was published in 1962. From its origins, initially with Professor Pickard at the helm, the subsequent editions have always promoted operative dentistry principles that placed tooth preservation first and foremost. Since this time there have been major advances in the science underpinning our subject. These include a better understanding of the complex pathological processes that cause hard tissue disease, along with its detection, diagnosis, and the operative technologies and adhesive/sealing dental materials used to manage the damaged tissues. This *minimally invasive* biologically based approach is now recognized as the gold standard, and we have embraced this with the change of book title of this current edition, to *Pickard's Guide to Minimally Invasive Operative Dentistry*.

The ninth edition received a major update in style and content based upon the sound foundations from its previous editions authored by Professors Smith and Kidd. In this new edition we have responded to reader feedback and have made the following changes:

- We have included a chapter on the principles of the operative management of the badly broken down tooth, leading the reader towards an appreciation of the intimate link between direct and indirect restorations.

- We have expanded the final chapter covering the long-term clinical management/maintenance of direct restorations, using the minimally invasive '5Rs' concept—*review, refurbish, reseal, repair*, and *replace*.

- With respect to referencing the information in the book, we felt that traditional reference lists at the end of each chapter become rapidly outdated in areas that are undergoing continuous evolution. Therefore in this edition we have introduced QR code images to allow the reader to access with their mobile devices original and supporting material resources through digital media. The use of keywords for searching online databases will allow the reader to review references that will evolve dynamically.

This edition has been significantly enhanced by the inclusion of more high-quality images to help illustrate scientific concepts and clinical scenarios. We must thank Dr Louis Mackenzie, who has kindly provided many of these additions. In addition, we wish to thank our many colleagues who have allowed us to use their illustrations. They are acknowledged in the captions to the relevant figures, together with the source of the original publication where applicable.

In the previous edition we reinforced the link between prevention, operative dentistry, and overall patient care. This *minimum intervention* care philosophy continues to underpin the current edition, with increasing emphasis placed upon the differing important roles of the oral healthcare team. The operative skill set of a new dental graduate has evolved to encompass not only the techniques, materials, and science of minimally invasive dentistry, but also, increasingly, the behaviour management of their patients. Without patients taking responsibility for their oral health, even the best operative dentistry will fail, regardless of the materials used. In this regard, the amalgam debate has not gone away. Indeed, as a result of the United Nations Minamata Treaty in 2013, the global environmental impact of dental amalgam has led to recommendations for a phase down in its clinical use. The treaty has highlighted the need for increased dental research into caries prevention and alternative restorative materials in conjunction with better professional education in their use. We sincerely hope that this book goes some way towards achieving the latter.

A.B.
T.F.W.
October 2014

Contents

1

Dental hard tissue pathologies, aetiology, and their clinical manifestations

Chapter contents

1.1 Introduction: why practise minimally invasive (tooth-preserving) operative dentistry?

Minimally invasive operative dentistry is that aspect of restorative dentistry which repairs and/or restores damaged and defective tooth structure directly in order to maintain pulp vitality, function, and aesthetics (see Figure 1.1). The primary goal is to respect tooth structure during this process, retaining viable and biologically repairable tissues to maintain tooth vitality for as long as possible. The hard tissue damage or defects can be caused by one or more of the following:

- caries
- tooth wear
- trauma
- developmental conditions.

Minimum intervention oral healthcare is that approach to patient management where the oral healthcare team (comprised of the dentist, nurses, oral health educators, hygienists, therapists, technicians, reception staff, and practice managers), led by the dentist, act as one to provide individualized patient-centred care and advice to encourage the patient to take responsibility for and maintain their own oral health. Minimum intervention care revolves around methods of detection/diagnosis/risk assessment of oral disease, non-operative control/prevention of these conditions, minimally invasive operative repair of tissue damage, and review/maintenance/recall of the patient and the advice/care offered by the dentist/team (see Figure 1.1). The process of care planning involves the patient, including disease prevention by behaviour change and adherence, not just listing those operative procedures offered to restore damaged or defective teeth in isolation. It must be understood from the outset that even though minimally invasive operative dentistry has a pivotal role in the 'surgical' repair of damaged teeth, it alone does not provide the actual cure for dental disease—please understand that '*drilling and filling teeth does not cure caries!*' The following sections will provide an overview of the four conditions mentioned previously with respect to their aetiology, histopathology, and microbiology where relevant. An attempt will be made to relate these features to the clinical manifestations of each condition, namely carious lesions and tooth-wear lesions.

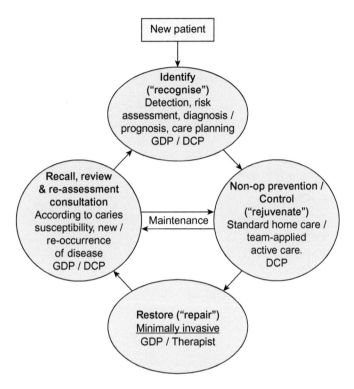

Figure 1.1 The patient-centred minimum intervention care cycle showing the four interlinking phases of patient assessment/diagnosis, non-operative prevention of lesions/control of disease, *minimally invasive* operative intervention, and review (recall). The arrows indicate the direction of patient flow through this cycle, and within each bubble an indication is given of the members of the dental team who might be included (GDP, general dental practitioner; DCP, dental care professional, including oral health educator-trained nurses, hygienists, therapists, practice managers, and reception staff).

1.2 Dental caries

1.2.1 What is it?

'A reversible (in its earliest stages) but progressive disease of the dental hard tissues, instigated by the action of bacteria upon fermentable carbohydrates in the plaque biofilm on tooth surfaces, leading to bacterially generated acid demineralization and ultimately proteolytic destruction of the organic component of the dental tissues.'

1.2.2 Terminology

Primary caries is the developing pathological biochemical process and physical lesion occurring on a previously sound tooth surface.

Root caries is primary caries on an exposed root surface (often after gingival recession has occurred), penetrating more easily into the exposed dentine. The pathological biochemical process for both primary and root caries is the same (see Figures 1.2 and 1.3).

Recurrent (secondary) caries is primary caries occurring at the margin of a failing restoration. An alternative definition of this is 'caries associated with restorations/sealants (CARS).' The aetiology is the same—metabolic activity in the stagnant plaque biofilm.

Residual caries is a term describing that portion of caries-affected, demineralized tissue retained purposely after minimally invasive cavity preparation, which is then sealed over and restored (see later).

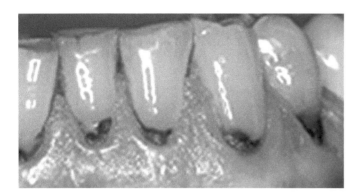

Figure 1.2 Slowly progressing root surface lesions with dark, leathery dentine surfaces and some plaque deposits. This is the mouth of a 70-year-old patient with a dry mouth (xerostomia, secondary Sjögren's syndrome) and rheumatoid arthritis, making oral hygiene difficult due to impaired toothbrush manipulation and painful mucosae.

1.2.3 Caries: the process and the lesion

The caries process

The caries process originates as metabolic activity in the plaque biofilm resident on the tooth surface. This biofilm begins to form just a few minutes after the tooth surface has been brushed, and is adsorbed initially as the *acquired pellicle* containing an admix of salivary proteins and glycoproteins. Within a short time, oral bacteria colonize the pellicle, thus forming the dental plaque biofilm, associated closely with bacterial extracellular polysaccharides and salivary proteins. The increased density of this developing biofilm, changing bacterial population, pH, and oxygen tension all combine to create a cariogenic environment on the tooth surface. This ubiquitous natural metabolic process cannot be prevented. However, disease progression can be *controlled* by the patient, with the help of the dentist and their oral healthcare team, so that a clinically visible enamel lesion never forms. The de- and remineralization metabolic processes can be modified, particularly by regular disturbance of the biofilm with a toothbrush and fluoride toothpaste. If the biofilm is partially or totally removed at regular close intervals, mineral loss may be stopped or even reversed towards mineral gain (especially in early or *incipient* lesions). The fluoride in toothpaste delays lesion progression primarily by inhibiting demineralization and encouraging remineralization processes.

The carious lesion

The carious lesion forms as a direct consequence of the metabolic activity in the biofilm on the tooth surface (i.e. the caries process). If factors tip the demineralization/remineralization balance towards demineralization (plaque, diet, salivary factors, mineral ion concentrations, and time), the histological stages of progressive lesion formation leading to cavitation can eventually be detected clinically and dealt with accordingly.

1.2.4 Aetiology of the caries process

Occurring in the plaque biofilm, the main factors that interact in the aetiology of the carious process are as follows:

- *Bacteria*: with colonization within the plaque biofilm, several hundred different species exist within a complex ecology, dependent on the age and relative stagnancy of the plaque on the tooth surface. *Streptococcus mutans*, classically thought to be the primary causative bacterial species, is now considered to have an associative role in the

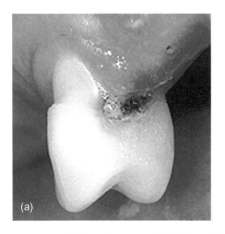
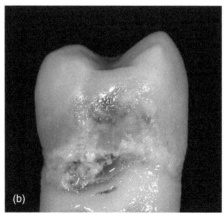
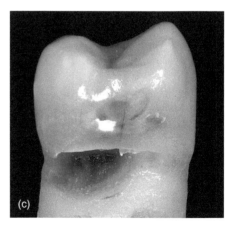

Figure 1.3 **(a)** An active root caries lesion with overlying plaque deposit in an area of stagnation alongside the margins of a partial denture. The buccal cervical abrasion cavity has been caused by excessive toothbrushing. **(b)** A stagnant plaque biofilm present on the proximal root surface, which when removed **(c)** reveals an active root caries lesion. (Images (b) and (c) courtesy of L. Mackenzie.)

Q1.1: What differences in clinical appearance are there between the coronal and root surface caries lesion in Figure 1.3 (c), and how may they relate to lesion activity?

caries process, and may act as a potential microbiological marker for caries. *Lactobacillus* and *Bifidobacterium* species have been shown to be significant in the caries process, and it is likely that species interaction within the biofilm will instigate and allow the carious lesion to progress.

- *Susceptible tooth surfaces* (see Chapter 2): carious lesions occur on tooth surfaces that have accumulated plaque, stagnating for a prolonged period of time, which may include the following:
  - The depths of pits and fissures on posterior occlusal/buccal surfaces of those teeth that the patient cannot clean effectively with a toothbrush. These areas on newly erupting molars are particularly susceptible to carious attack.
  - Proximal surfaces (mesial and distal) *cervical* to the contact points of adjacent teeth (where the patient may not floss regularly, or at all). These surfaces of particularly imbricated (crowded) teeth can be more susceptible due to the lack of access for oral hygiene aids.
  - Smooth surfaces adjacent to the gingival margin (again an area that the patient may often miss with their toothbrush), especially of those teeth that are imbricated, rotated or in-standing.
  - The ledged/overhanging/defective margins of restorations (a plaque trap created, often not evident to the patient, and inaccessible to a toothbrush or floss) (see Figure 1.4).
- *Fermentable carbohydrates*: plaque bacteria are capable of metabolizing certain dietary carbohydrates (including sucrose and glucose), producing various organic acids (lactic, acetic, and propionic acids) at the tooth surface, causing plaque pH to fall within 1–3 minutes, and initiating demineralization if the pH drops to below 5.5 (critical pH of enamel). The pH can take up to 60 minutes to climb back to normal levels, this normalization being aided by the protective buffering capacity of saliva (pH 7.0; see Figure 1.5). This demineralization/remineralization cycle occurs continuously at any tooth surface, all the time.
- *Time*: even though the drop in pH commences rapidly, sufficient time is required for the plaque biofilm to produce a *net* mineral loss equating to histological hard tissue damage at the tooth surface.

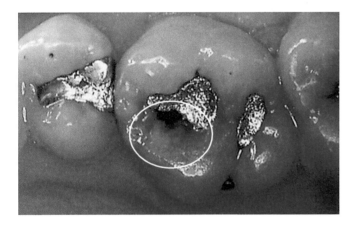

Figure 1.4 Caries at the margin of the failed dental amalgam restoration (white circle) on the occlusal surface of UL6.

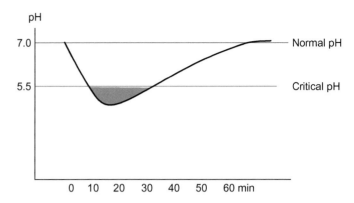

Figure 1.5 The Stephan curve, showing the changes in plaque pH over time after an oral glucose rinse at time 0 minutes. The critical pH of enamel (5.5) is that below which the hydroxyapatite crystals begin to dissociate into their constituent ions. Note that the critical pH varies, depending on an inversely proportional correlation with the concentration of available calcium and phosphate ions in the plaque biofilm fluid at the tooth surface. The grey-shaded portion of the graph indicates the 20-minute period in which the tooth surface is under threat of mineral loss. The critical pH of dentine is 6.2, which again is not fixed.

The four direct causes previously discussed can be affected or modified by several other indirect patient factors to affect ultimately the disease pattern experienced by each individual patient. These determinants include the patient's:

- income (the cost of dental care)
- knowledge about their own oral health
- attitudes to healthcare (general and oral)
- social class
- behaviour
- education.

The relative importance of these factors can be determined during verbal history taking (anamnesis) and oral examination (see Chapter 2), and helps to form the basis for determining the individual's risk and likelihood of developing caries in the future—the caries risk assessment/likelihood analysis (see Chapter 3). It is these factors in combination with the collective skills of the oral healthcare team that will help the patient to overcome or 'cure' their condition of dental caries.

1.2.5 Speed and severity of the caries process

The caries process in the normal oral environment, whose metabolic activity is tipped in favour of demineralization, will take several weeks to become detectable clinically as a lesion with signs and symptoms. This is because the overall process, with its continuously fluctuating metabolic balance at the ionic level, is relatively slow and can be moderated by oral hygiene techniques, dietary modification, and the use of fluoride or other agents. The presence of saliva, with its capacity to buffer plaque acids, provide a source of remineralizing calcium and phosphate ions to the tooth/lesion surface, remove food debris, and lubricate/protect tooth surfaces, also helps.

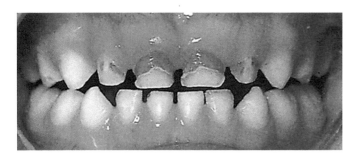

Figure 1.6 Early childhood caries affecting deciduous anterior teeth.

Q1.2: What habit(s) may have contributed to this pattern of disease?

'Rampant' caries

However, clinical scenarios exist where the process is accelerated and many biochemically active lesions form rapidly, often involving surfaces of teeth ordinarily expected to be caries-free—described classically as 'rampant' caries. This condition affects the primary dentition, where it is now more appropriately termed *early childhood caries* (see Figure 1.5), teenagers, or young adults with a highly cariogenic diet (frequent sugar episodes; see Figure 1.6) and/or addicted to recreational drugs, or adult patients with a dry mouth (xerostomia) (see Figure 1.7). Radiation to the region of the salivary glands, used in the treatment of an orofacial malignant growth, and Sjögren's syndrome, an autoimmune condition that may involve the salivary glands, are the most common causes of severe xerostomia. In addition, a large number of therapeutic drugs, such as antidepressants, tranquillizers, antihypertensive drugs, and diuretics can retard salivary flow and affect its quality, especially when taken together (polypharmacy).

Arrested caries

In distinct contrast to rampant caries, the term *arrested caries* describes those lesions that have stopped progressing and are inactive

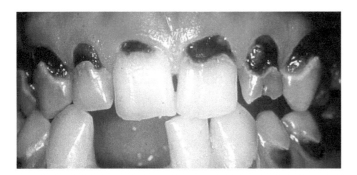

Figure 1.7 Rampant caries in an adult patient with cavities affecting sites not normally associated with caries due to their accessibility for adequate oral hygiene.

Q1.3: What aetiological factors may have contributed to this pattern of disease?

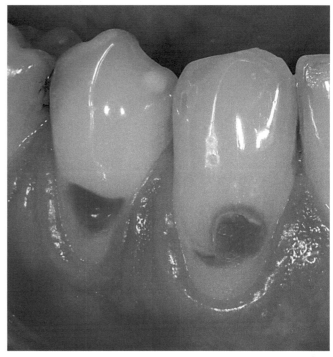

Figure 1.8 A hard, shiny, and stained arrested root surface lesion is present on the buccal cervical aspect of the LR4. However, the lesion on the LR3 has a matte, stippled surface appearance indicative of lesion activity. (Courtesy of L. Mackenzie.)

Q1.4: Why might the lesion on the LR3 appear active whereas the adjacent lesion on the LR4 in the same patient appears arrested?

metabolically. It is observed when factors in the oral environment have changed from conditions predisposing to caries to conditions that tend to slow, or even reverse, lesion progression. These 'arrested' lesions often have a dark, hard, shiny exposed dentine surface (see Figure 1.8 and Table 1.1).

1.2.6 The carious lesion

Having summarized the caries process as an ongoing metabolic demineralization/remineralization balance occurring at the interface between the plaque biofilm and the tooth surface, it is important to understand that the resulting carious lesion is a progressive alteration and destruction of the hard tissues (mineral and organic matrix) from the enamel surface through to the pulp. While the lesion is still within enamel, it can be arrested and possibly reversed with net mineral gain in its earliest stages. Once it is into dentine, the process can be made inactive (arrested), but if proteolytic destruction of the organic collagen matrix has occurred extensively, this cannot be reversed as observed histologically. This section will take the reader through key features of the histological and clinical development of a lesion from its earliest enamel stages through to cavitation into the pulp.

An understanding of the basic histological features of healthy enamel and dentine is an essential prerequisite for appreciating the changes

Table 1.1 Summary of differences in physical characteristics between active and inactive (arrested) carious lesions in enamel or dentine

	Physical characteristics of the carious lesion	
	Active	Inactive (arrested)
Enamel	Surface of enamel is white/yellow; opaque with loss of lustre; feels rough when the tip of the ball-ended probe is moved gently across the surface. Lesion is in a plaque stagnation area (i.e. pits and fissures), or near the gingival and proximal surface below the contact point. Lesion covered by plaque biofilm prior to examination (WSL)	Surface of enamel is whitish, brownish, or black. Enamel is shiny and feels hard and smooth when the tip of the ball-ended probe is moved gently across the surface. For smooth surfaces, the lesion is typically located at some distance from the gingival margin. Lesion not covered by plaque prior to examination (BSL)
Dentine	Dentine appears moist and matte; feels rough, soft, and wet or leathery on gentle probing	Dentine appears shiny and hard, and is scratchy on gentle probing

WSL, white spot lesion; BSL, brown spot lesion.

that occur within the lesion, and an outline of these is presented in Table 7.1 in Chapter 7. Further information can be obtained from the suggested further reading at the end of this chapter. The relationship between lesion histology and clinical appearance has been used in a caries detection and assessment system which is outlined and discussed in Chapter 2 (see Table 2.3).

Within enamel

Plaque-acid demineralization causes porosities to form within the prism structure, initially beneath the outer surface of enamel: this is termed *subsurface demineralization*. The developing pore volumes through the depth of the enamel lesion, caused by a longer exposure to reduced pH, have been measured using polarized light microscopy (outermost surface zone (< 1% pore volume), body (5–25%), dark (2–4%), and innermost translucent zone (1%); see Figure 1.9).

The existence of the enamel lesion surface zone may be due to increased extrinsic fluoride ion deposition in this area, or as a consequence of remineralization metabolism of the biofilm on the tooth surface. It is essential that this intact surface is not cavitated iatrogenically (i.e. a hole created by a dentist/therapist sticking a sharp dental probe/explorer into the lesion surface; see Chapter 2, Figure 2.7), as it still has the potential to heal if the biofilm can be regularly and effectively removed by the patient, and remineralizing solutions and/or toothpastes containing higher concentrations of calcium and phosphate ions used periodically (see Chapter 4, Section 4.2.3).

Histologically, smooth surface lesions have a cross-sectional shape of an inverted cone (widest superficially, with the apex towards the

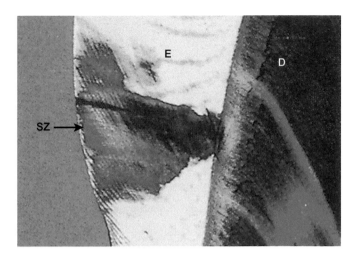

Figure 1.9 Longitudinal ground section through a carious lesion on a smooth surface (polarized light and water; E, enamel; D, dentine). The enamel lesion is shaped as an inverted cone, widest at the tooth surface, narrowing towards the enamel–dentine junction, with a relatively intact surface zone (SZ).

Q1.5: What ions have contributed to the creation of the intact surface zone and where have they come from?

enamel–dentine junction (EDJ); see Figure 1.10). Fissure lesions can be considered to take the form of two adjacent smooth surface lesions (see Figure 1.11).

- *Clinical manifestations* (see Table 1.1): the active white spot lesion (WSL) is initially smooth, frosty white/opaque, and non-cavitated

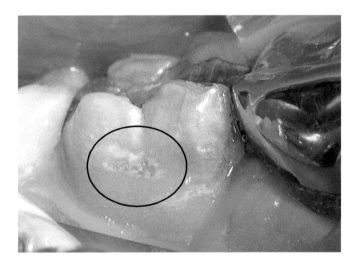

Figure 1.10 Active white spot enamel lesion on the mid-buccal of LL7 (circled). This more developed lesion has a rough surface, acting as a plaque trap.

Q1.6: What features of the lesion in Figure 1.10 will help the dentist to conclude that it is active, how might these be detected, and how might the patient be managed?

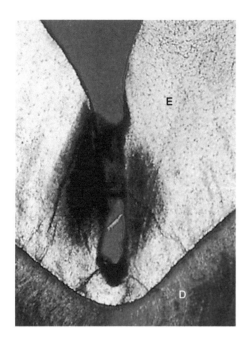

Figure 1.11 A longitudinal ground section (polarized light with water) through an occlusal fissure showing an enamel lesion forming on the two adjacent walls of the fissure (dark regions; E, enamel; D, dentine).

Q1.7: How might this scenario be managed in a high caries risk patient?

---

clinically (see Figure 1.12). This can be detected more easily if the tooth surface is air-dried for a few seconds using a 3-1 air/water syringe. As the lesion develops over time, it becomes somewhat chalky, eventually becoming roughened or micro-cavitated (roughness can be detected by gently running a rounded/ball-ended probe *across* the lesion surface). This surface irregularity can encourage further plaque deposition (see Figure 1.10). There are no symptoms at this stage, but reactions in the dentine–pulp complex may be mediated by cytokines and bacterial breakdown products within the dentine matrix and tubules (see later).

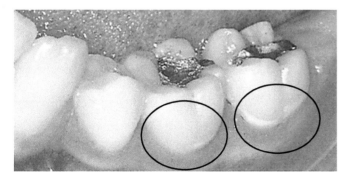

Figure 1.12 Early white spot enamel lesions on the cervical-gingival margins of both mandibular left molars (circled).

If plaque is removed, these lesions can arrest and porosities can be eliminated by abrasive toothbrushing/tooth wear, resulting in the hard smooth shiny surfaces of arrested lesions. Porosities may also be filled with deposited mineral and dietary molecules causing staining (e.g. tannins), which may be trapped within the mineral lattice. This process creates an arrested brown spot lesion (BSL) with a hard shiny overlying smooth surface (see Figure 1.13b).

The lesion at the EDJ or the amelo–dentinal junction (ADJ)

Histologically, the caries process may reach dentine before clinical cavitation is detectable (a closed lesion: mICDAS score 2; see Chapter 2). Defence reactions in the dentine–pulp complex are stimulated at this stage, with evidence of translucent dentine at the advancing lesion boundary and tertiary dentine deposition at the dentine–pulp interface beneath the advancing lesion (see later). Again, symptoms are unlikely at this stage of lesion development.

The lesion extends in dentine, immediately subjacent to the EDJ (see Figure 1.13a), its lateral extension coinciding with the spread of the overlying enamel lesion at the surface of the tooth, which in turn is dependent on the extent of the resident plaque biofilm at the tooth surface. Relative hypomineralization of this histological mantle dentine zone, greater side-branching of dentine tubules, or defects within the enamel/dentine interface may also contribute to this spread laterally.

The lesion may also penetrate along the dentine tubules towards the pulp.

Within dentine

Once the lesion has spread histologically (and radiographically) further towards the middle third of dentine, it is often cavitated (open) clinically on both occlusal and smooth surfaces, with plaque now able to accumulate on the exposed dentine surface. The further spread of the lesion will undermine the overlying enamel, creating an associated visible grey shadow/opacity, which becomes brittle and prone to fracture under occlusal loading. This undermined and unsupported enamel may need to be removed during cavity preparation if the damage requires operative repair (see Chapter 5, Section 5.9.3).

The patient may begin to experience initial symptoms of acute pulpitis—a poorly localized sharp pain of a few seconds' duration stimulated by hot, cold, or sweet stimuli (see Chapter 3). The histological components of carious dentine to be considered are the mineral, collagen, bacterial penetration, and tubule structure. Both degenerative and reparative processes act on these simultaneously in different parts of the lesion. The histological changes of the carious dentine biomass through its depth (from EDJ to pulp) are described in the following bullet points, but note that these descriptive zones are not separate biological entities, but blend into one another without clear detectable boundaries (see Figure 1.14).

- *Caries-infected dentine* (zone 1 in Figure 1.14): the outermost, superficial, irreparable, necrotic zone of destruction, often distinguished clinically as a dark brown, soft, wet, 'mushy' layer.
  - Mineral component has dissociated extensively due to bacterial acid attack.

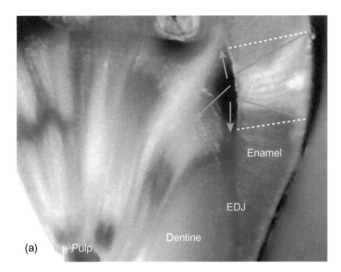
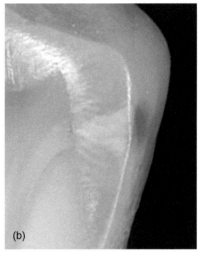

Figure 1.13 (a) A mesio-distal section through a carious tooth highlighting a proximal lesion. The red lines outline the 'inverted cone' cross-sectional histological shape of the enamel lesion, and the blue arrows indicate the direction of spread of the lesion having crossed the enamel–dentine junction (EDJ) into dentine. The white dotted lines show how the extent of the spread of the dentine lesion subjacent to the EDJ is associated with the same lateral extent of the enamel lesion on the tooth surface, both governed by the presence of the plaque biofilm at the tooth surface. (b) The surface lesion shown is an arrested brown spot lesion, its boundaries clearly aligned with the inverted cone of the enamel lesion beneath. (Figure 1.13 (b) courtesy of L. Mackenzie.)

Q1.8: How will the patient have arrested this once active lesion?

- Collagenous matrix has been denatured (irreparably damaged) by proteolytic enzymes intrinsic to the dentine itself (the zinc-dependent, acid-activated matrix metalloproteinases (MMPs)), as well as from bacteria, activated by those bacterial acids produced during the caries process.
- Bacterial load in this zone is very high.
- Dentine tubule structure is destroyed.

This zone of 'necrotic' dentine should be clinically removed when preparing a cavity, as it cannot be repaired histologically and it provides a poor-quality bonding substrate for adhesive materials to achieve an adequate seal, and inadequate physical restoration support.

- *Caries-affected dentine* (zones 2, 3, and 4 combined together; see Figure 1.14): the inner layer of carious dentine which can be repaired by the dentine–pulp complex, often distinguished as paler brown, harder, 'sticky and scratchy', or slightly leathery dentine (elicited by a sharp dental probe, which should not be used directly over the pulpal floor of a deep cavity).
  - Mineral dissolution still occurs, but to a lesser extent than in infected dentine, as the pH gradually rises towards the advancing front of the lesion and the ionic equilibrium begins to balance.
  - Collagen is still damaged by proteolysis, but to a lesser extent, so permitting dentine repair/mineral gain, as the proteinaceous scaffold for mineral crystal deposition now persists.

- Bacterial load lessens, but there are still more anaerobic bacteria present.
- Dentine tubule structure returns gradually within the depths of this zone.

The deepest layer of caries-affected dentine (zone 4 in Figure 1.14) can be described as hypermineralized translucent dentine (due to its glassy appearance in histological cross-section), one of several reparative reactions of the dentine–pulp complex to the caries process (see later). As can be seen in Figures 1.13 and 1.14, the lesion in dentine often has a dark brown discoloration within the caries-infected zone which then pales gradually through the depth of the lesion, towards the pulp. The aetiology of the colour changes is not clear, but a biochemical reaction between proteins and carbohydrates in a moist acidic biological environment, the *Maillard reaction*, may play a part. Not all lesions are uniformly dark brown; some rapidly advancing lesions may have a pale discoloration within the caries-infected zone, and there is no direct link between the colour of dentine and the bacteria present within these zones.

1.2.7 Carious pulp exposure

If the carious process cannot be modified by preventive or controlling measures and the lesion is not treated operatively in time with appropriate minimally invasive excavation techniques and a sealed adhesive restoration within the dentine, then the advancing front of the lesion will approach the dentine–pulp boundary. By this point, bacteria/toxins

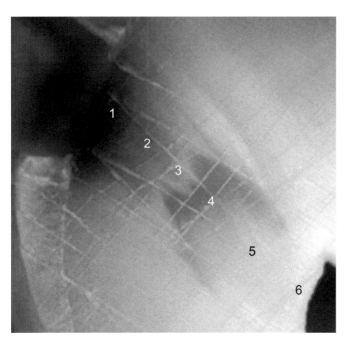

Figure 1.14 A mesio-distal section through a proximal lesion showing a cavity in the enamel and the histological colour changes through the dentine lesion (1, caries-infected dentine; 2, 3, and 4, caries-affected dentine; 4, translucent dentine; 5, 6, sound dentine). The surface criss-cross scratches were placed to act as reference markers during microscopy analysis of the sample.

Q1.9: What are the potential causes of the colour change in dentine caries?

will have penetrated into the pulp tissues causing an acute inflammatory response. Depending on the timescale over which this has happened, an initial acute pulpitic response (poorly localized short, sharp pain on exposure to hot, cold, or sweet stimuli) will evolve into a more chronic response, changing the symptoms experienced towards a dull, prolonged ache that may last for several minutes and is spontaneous and non-specific in origin (see Chapter 3). The cavity will probably have enlarged due to the undermined enamel having been broken away (including the marginal ridges of proximal lesions) during function, and will be noticeable to the patient as 'a hole in the tooth' or 'cavity.'

If the pulp chamber is breached physically by the lesion, a *carious exposure* may be created when excavating deep caries, and the exposed pulp tissue will bleed uncontrollably for several minutes before cotton wool pledgets can achieve haemostasis. In most cases of a carious pulp exposure, root canal treatment is the management option of choice (as long as the tooth is restorable with a worthwhile prognosis), but this will depend on the size of the exposure, the age of the patient (a young, well-vascularized pulp may have a better prognosis), and the severity of the carious process within the depth of the lesion (see Chapter 5). In rare cases, on late presentation, the pulp soft tissues undergo a hyperplastic cellular reaction and appear to herniate through the exposure, into the cavity.

If minimally invasive excavation principles and techniques are used to excavate carefully the deeper aspects of the carious lesion, the risk of a carious exposure is reduced (see Chapter 5). In cases where the pulp is deemed vital on initial clinical examination, it may be appropriate best practice to retain caries-affected dentine as an 'indirect pulp cap', sealing the cavity with a suitable long-term adhesive restoration and then reviewing the pulp status at subsequent planned recall appointments. Several clinical studies have shown this to be an effective minimally invasive method for maintaining the pulp vitality of teeth, so reducing the need for root canal treatment (see later).

1.2.8 Dentine–pulp complex reparative reactions

Dentine is a vital tissue containing the cytoplasmic extensions of odontoblasts, and must be considered together with the pulp, since the two tissues are so intimately connected. The dentine–pulp complex, like any other vital tissue in the body, is capable of defending itself. The state of the tissue at any time will depend on the balance between the attacking forces and the defence reactions. The defence reactions include deposition of *translucent dentine*, *tertiary dentine*, and *pulpal inflammation*.

Translucent dentine

Sometimes incorrectly referred to as 'sclerotic' dentine, this glassy zone of dentine (zone 4 in Figure 1.14) is caused by tubular infill with plate-like Whitlockite mineral crystals (β-octocalciumphosphate) at the advancing front of the lesion in an attempt to wall off the advancing lesion. Its appearance is due to the parity of refractive indices of intertubular and intratubular mineral, so allowing light to pass through the sectioned boundaries.

The Whitlockite deposits originate from a combination of a physico-chemical re-precipitation of calcium and phosphate ions diffusing towards the increasing pH environment of the lesion's deepest advancing front, and also possibly a vital process of new and rapid mineral deposition from the pulp via the odontoblasts. Even though hypermineralized, this zone of translucent dentine is softer than its deeper, sound counterpart due to the weaker crystalline orientation of Whitlockite than conventional hydroxyapatite crystals within the tubules (analogous to stacking dinner plates flat—too tall a stack and they topple over!) (see Figure 1.15).

Tertiary (reactionary/reparative/irritation/atubular) dentine

Secondary dentine is laid down throughout life as part of the normal pulp–dentine complex (see Figure 1.16). Tertiary dentine is laid down at the dentine–pulp border in response to a noxious stimulus (e.g. caries or those causing tooth wear), in an attempt to wall off and distance the pulp from the advancing noxious stimulus (see Figure 1.17). It may resemble secondary dentine histologically, but has an irregular tubular or atubular structure, depending on the speed of its creation. *Reactionary dentine* (see Figure 1.18) is deposited as a result of a mild irritant where original odontoblasts survive and are metabolically up-regulated. *Reparative dentine* (see Figure 1.19) is much more irregular and is deposited in response to a stronger irritant which compromises the vitality of the original odontoblasts. Progenitor cells from the sub-odontoblastic layer then differentiate and are up-regulated to produce an atubular defence reaction.

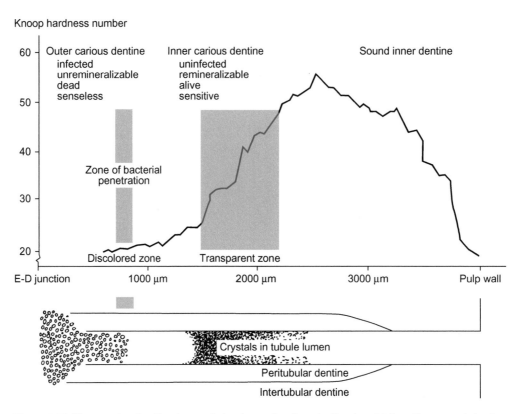

Figure 1.15 Diagram showing the changes in hardness of carious dentine (y-axis) from the enamel–dentine junction (EDJ) towards the pulp (x-axis), and relating this to the histological changes that occur through the dentine lesion. The transparent zone (synonymous with the translucent zone) is softer than the deeper, less mineralized, sound dentine. The diagram equates the bacterial content and mineral deposition within the tubule lumen through the progressive zones of carious dentine. Reproduced from O Fejerskov and E Kidd. *Dental Caries – the disease and its clinical management.* Copyright © 2008, John Wiley and Sons Ltd.)

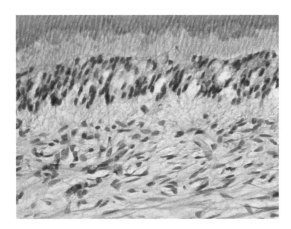

Figure 1.16 Haematoxylin and eosin (H&E) section of normal dentine–pulp complex with pale pink stained pre-dentine zone visible at the top of the image. This will undergo mineralization as part of the normal ageing process, as secondary dentine is laid down in the pulp chamber. (Courtesy of Carlos A. de Souza Costa.)

Q1.10: Can you identify two cellular zones in the pulp (the cell nuclei are stained purple)?

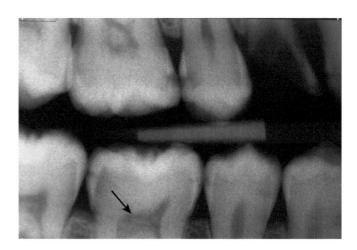

Figure 1.17 Right bitewing radiograph of a patient with high caries rate and multiple lesions. Note the dentine–pulp complex reparative response of LR6 to the distal dentine lesion—the distal pulp horn has been obliterated by deposits of tertiary dentine (arrow).

Q1.11: How many other carious lesions can you detect?

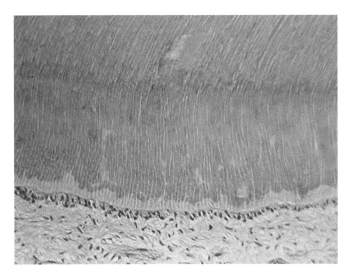

Figure 1.18 H&E section of pulp–dentine complex showing *reactionary dentine* in the middle of the field of view. (Courtesy of Carlos A. de Souza Costa.)

Q1.12: Can you identify five histological zones in the H&E section in Figure 1.18 from top to bottom?

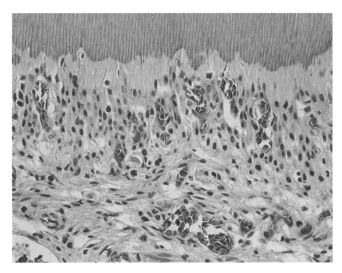

Figure 1.19 H&E section of pulp–dentine complex showing *reparative dentine*, along with the associated, disorganized, and newly differentiated odontoblasts. In the middle of the field of view can be seen bright red blood cells, associated with the pulp's inflammatory response. (Courtesy of Carlos A. de Souza Costa.)

Pulp inflammation

This is the fundamental response of all vascular connective tissues to injury. Inflammation of the pulp (pulpitis) may, as in any other tissue, be acute or chronic. In a slowly progressing carious lesion, toxins reaching the pulp may provoke chronic inflammation. However, once the organisms actually reach the pulp (a carious exposure), acute inflammation may supervene. Inflammatory reactions have vascular and cellular components. In chronic inflammation the cellular components predominate and there may be increased collagen production, leading to fibrosis, but without immediately endangering the vitality of the tooth. However, in acute inflammation the vascular changes predominate.

Infection is the most common cause of pulp inflammation, and caries is the most common microbial source. Dentine caries will result

in pulp inflammation, and chronic inflammatory cells (macrophages, lymphocytes, and plasma cells) will infiltrate the pulp near the odontoblast layer. Indeed, this infiltration has been detected in response to initial enamel caries. This chronic inflammatory reaction is due mainly to the movement of bacterial toxins through the dentine tubules. Secretory immunoglobulins travel in the dentine fluid up the remaining patent tubules. With increasing carious involvement of enamel and dentine, the area of chronic inflammation increases in size, but it is believed to remain localized until pulp exposure. Bacteria may enter the pulp with polymorphonuclear leucocytes predominating, and acute inflammation can supervene, spread throughout the pulp, and result in necrosis.

1.3 Tooth wear ('tooth surface loss')

Tooth wear (TW) is 'the irreversible surface loss of dental hard tissues caused by factors other than caries or trauma.' It can be physiological, occurring slowly and naturally throughout life, or pathological, occurring at a much faster rate, usually caused by combinations of erosion, attrition, abrasion, and perhaps abfraction (see Table 1.2).

Erosion can be defined as the irreversible loss of dental hard tissues by a chemical process (acid attack) not involving bacteria. It is often the common denominator in the multifactorial aetiology of tooth wear. Sources of acid can be either intrinsic (stomach acid regurgitation) or extrinsic (dietary, environmental). Involuntary gastro-oesophageal reflux disease (GORD) is a common cause of intrinsic stomach acids entering the oral cavity on a regular basis, and occurs primarily due to transient relaxation or incompetence of the lower oesophageal

sphincter. Certain factors in combination often predispose to GORD, and these factors may include:

- diet—fatty, spicy foods consumed in large quantities, especially late at night
- alcohol
- certain medications (e.g. diazepam)
- causes of increased gastric pressure, including obesity, pregnancy, posture (lying down increases pressure on the sphincter), and even excessive exercise
- gastro-oesophageal reflux predisposes to further GORD symptoms
- neuromuscular conditions.

Table 1.2 Tooth wear: common aetiology, features, and simple classification

Aetiological factors		Comments
Erosion	Intrinsic, regurgitation (GORD*, vomiting)	Common cause of erosion; affects palatal surfaces of maxillary anterior teeth, occlusal/buccal surfaces of lower molars. Stomach hydrochloric acid originates from: • involuntary GORD • involuntary/voluntary vomiting
	Extrinsic, dietary	Affects labial surfaces of maxillary anterior teeth. ⊠ pH due to excess acidic food/drink intake: • citrus fruit and fruit juices • pickles, vinegar-containing foodstuffs • carbonated drinks (including diet/health drinks) • some mouthwashes have a low pH Drinking habits: through straw and frothing around mouth. Acids include citric, carbonic, acetic, hydrochloric, and phosphoric acids. Often associated with a healthy lifestyle—patient understanding is required to modify the erosive potential of the diet
	Extrinsic, environmental	Labial surfaces of maxillary anteriors/pitting. Rare nowadays due to stringent health and safety regulations in the workplace. Historically caused by industrial processes where acid was vaporized and inhaled (battery manufacturers, tanning factories)
Attrition		TW caused by occlusal tooth–tooth contact; occlusal facets match with opposing teeth; usually in combination with erosion. Often caused by grinding/parafunctional habits
Abrasion		TW caused by tooth–non-tooth contact; hard toothbrushing with coarse toothpastes, dish-/V-shaped, smooth cervical lesions; incisal wear/grooves from long-term habitual behaviour (e.g. pipe smokers, milliners holding pins between their teeth, builders holding nails between their teeth, etc.)
Abfraction		Cervical V-shaped enamel–dentine TW lesions with no history of abrasion. Aetiology not clear, but masticatory stresses may concentrate at cervical margins of teeth and perhaps open up pre-existing cracks/weaknesses in the tooth

*GORD, gastro-oesophageal reflux disease.

Treatment for GORD will depend on the aetiology. As well as conservative management involving modifying diet, lifestyle, and the use of chewing gums, stomach acids can be neutralized using conventional antacids (e.g. Gaviscon), or their production limited with oral medications, including proton pump inhibitors (e.g. omeprazole (Losec)) or H_2 antagonists (e.g. cimetidine). Surgical procedures can be performed to repair physical damage to the gastro-oesophageal system. Once this has been done, any dental damage can be repaired. The patient's dentist may often be the first to notice the problem through the dental manifestations, and appropriate referral to medical colleagues may be required.

Intrinsic acids can also enter the oral cavity through voluntary or involuntary vomiting, causes of which may be:

• psychosomatic:
  ◦ eating disorders:
    (a) bulimia nervosa (affects 1–2% of the adolescent population; female:male ratio is 10:1)
    (b) anorexia nervosa (affects 0.1–1% of the teenage population; female:male ratio is 10:1)
  ◦ rumination (voluntary regurgitation followed by re-digestion of stomach contents)
  ◦ stress-induced psychogenic vomiting
• metabolic/endocrine:
  ◦ pregnancy
• gastrointestinal disorders:
  ◦ peptic ulcer/gastritis
  ◦ hiatus hernia
  ◦ achalasia—a condition associated with a narrowed lower oesophageal sphincter and reduced oesophageal motility, leading to stagnation and fermentation of ingested food within the oesophagus, and concomitant regurgitation
  ◦ cerebral palsy
• drug induced:
  ◦ primary—cytotoxic drugs
  ◦ secondary—gastric irritation, alcohol, aspirin, and other non-steroidal anti-inflammatory medications.

Again, in all of the cases listed, the initial cause of the vomiting must be found out from the patient's history and examination, and the cause itself treated first, with close cooperation with the patient's medical practitioner, before restoring any damaged dentition (see Chapter 2).

The aetiology and features of abrasion and attrition have been outlined in Table 1.2. Patients suffering from dry mouth with reduced and/or chemically or physically altered saliva may also be more at risk from dental erosion. This is because they will lack the protective features of saliva, which include the ability to neutralize/buffer intra-oral acids and to supply mineral ions for potential mineral deposition, including statherins and proline-rich proteins. The mucin component of saliva may also help to protect the tooth surfaces from dietary acids, with contributions to the formation of the surface pellicle and biofilm. Erosion is often a contributory factor in the overall pattern of clinical tooth wear. Acid-softened tooth surfaces are more susceptible to long-term 'wear' forces from opposing teeth (attrition) or other external influences (abrasion). Clinical examples of these are shown in Chapter 2.

1.4 Dental trauma

Whereas caries and tooth wear are diseases of relatively slow onset, traumatic injuries are acquired suddenly, and when these involve the hard dental tissues and the pulp they usually require immediate operative management to stabilize the condition, provide pain relief, and restore function and appearance if possible. Trauma to the mouth can produce any combination of the following local injuries:

- lacerations to the lips, tongue, and buccal and gingival tissue
- alveolar fractures, so that a number of teeth become mobile within a block of bone
- complete or partial subluxation of a tooth
- root fracture
- damage to the apical blood vessels without fracture
- fracture of the crown of the tooth involving enamel alone, enamel and dentine, or exposure of the pulp (see Figure 2.25 in Chapter 2).

1.4.1 Aetiology

Trauma is commonly caused by the following:

- falls
- sports/athletics injuries
- blows from a heavy object
- fights
- car/bicycle accidents
- injuries sustained during convulsive seizures (e.g. epilepsy)
- battered child syndrome (the most difficult and yet the most important cause to diagnose).

Detection and management will be discussed in subsequent chapters. Examples of dental trauma can be seen in Figures 1.20 and 1.21.

In some cases, untreated traumatic injury can lead to the development of long-term pathology (see Figure 1.21).

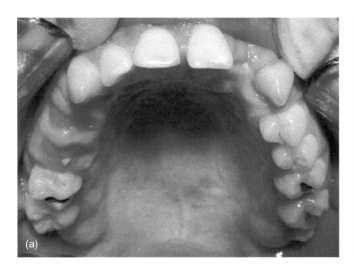
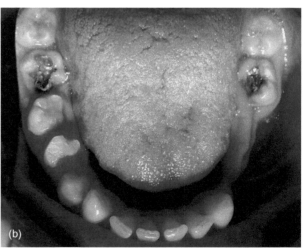

Figure 1.20 a, b Maxillary and mandibular occlusal views of a patient who has sustained multiple facial blows in a fight. Note the decoronated UR4,5 and large enamel and dentine fractures sustained on UR6, UL7, LR4,5,6, and LL6. UL2 and LL45 were avulsed in the incident.

Q1.13: What might have been the presenting dental complaints for the patient in Figure 1.20?

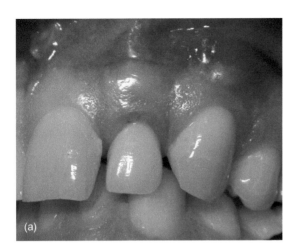

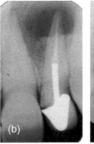 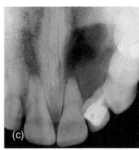 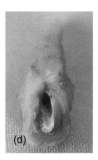

Figure 1.21 **(b)** Periapical and **(c)** upper standard occlusal (USO) radiographs of the UL123 shown in **(a)**. Note the large well-demarcated pathological radiolucency originating from the root apex of the fractured and displaced root, post-core, and crown complex in the UL2. The lesion is tracking in the overlying mucosa to the swelling pointed out in **(a)**. **(d)** The extracted UL2 root with the post-core and crown removed, showing the crack sustained from the impact.

Figure 1.21 **(a)** A fit and well young adult has sustained an accidental blow to the teeth in the UL123 area several months earlier.

Q1.14: Can you detect any abnormal clinical findings from Figure 1.21 (clue—check the mucosae)?

Q1.15: What other findings are evident from the USO radiograph?

1.5 Developmental defects

Teeth do not always develop normally, and there are a number of defects in tooth structure or shape which occur during development and become apparent on eruption. Such teeth are often unsightly or prone to excessive tooth wear or loss of clinical crowns, and thus they may require restoration to improve appearance or function or to protect the underlying tooth structure. These defects, their aetiology, and their clinical appearance are outlined in Table 2.7 in Chapter 2, with examples shown, and they include the acquired conditions of enamel hypoplasia, molar–incisor hypomineralization and intrinsic staining (fluorosis and tetracycline), as well as the hereditary conditions of hypodontia, amelogenesis imperfecta, and dentinogenesis imperfecta.

1.6 Suggested further reading and PubMed keywords

Fejerskov O and Kidd E A M (eds) (2008) *Dental Caries: the disease and its clinical management*. Oxford: Blackwell Munksgaard.
<http://eu.wiley.com/WileyCDA/WileyTitle/productCd1405138890,descCd-tableOfContents.html>

<www.ncbi.nlm.nih.gov/pubmed/advanced>

QR code image 1.1 Try searching the following keywords on PubMed for relevant further reading. You can access PubMed by scanning the QR code image or at the address

Keywords

Sjögren's syndrome; xerostomia; Maillard reaction and caries; dentine matrix metalloproteinases (MMPs); tooth wear; GORD and dental symptoms; hereditary dental conditions.

 1.7 Answers to self-test questions

Q1.1: What differences in clinical appearance are there between the coronal and root surface caries lesion in Figure 1.3c, and how may they relate to lesion activity?
A: See Table 1.1.

Q1.2: What habit(s) may have contributed to this pattern of disease?
A: This child was allowed to suck a bottle of sweet drink frequently.

Q1.3: What aetiological factors may have contributed to this pattern of disease?

A: If you look closely at the lesion on LR3, you will notice an undermined periphery of enamel. Plaque stagnation has occurred beneath this rim, so activating the lesion metabolically.

Q1.4: Why might the lesion on the LR3 appear active whereas the adjacent lesion on the LR4 in the same patient appears arrested?

A: Improved oral hygiene would have arrested this active part of the lesion.

Q1.5: What ions have contributed to the creation of the intact surface zone and where have they come from?

A: Fluoride, calcium, and phosphate ions in particular help to form a more acid-resistant fluoride-substituted hydroxyapatite. These ions will have come from the saliva as well as from the biofilm, in higher concentrations, so creating a positive equilibrium with the tooth surface.

Q1.6: What features of the lesion in Figure 1.10 will help the dentist to conclude that it is active, how might these be detected, and how might the patient be managed?

A: The lesion has surface roughness (detectable as vibrations in the handle of the ball-ended explorer as it is gently run across the lesion surface) and was covered with plaque (detected visually with a disclosing agent). This patient was under preventive therapy, including modifications of their oral hygiene, possibly diet, and application of fluoride varnish to arrest the lesion.

Q1.7: How might this scenario be managed in a high caries risk patient?

A: Instruct the patient regarding their oral hygiene procedures, and if this does not improve then carry out debridement/air abrasion followed by application of a fissure sealant.

Q1.8: How will the patient have arrested this once active lesion?

A: They will have done so by judiciously removing the plaque biofilm regularly using proper oral hygiene methods, including floss. This combined with the use of a fluoride dentifrice, over time, will inactivate the incipient WSL into the brown spot lesion seen in the image.

Q1.9: What are the potential causes of the colour change in dentine caries?

A: Although not conclusive, this may be due to the Maillard reaction—a biochemical reaction between proteins and carbohydrates in a moist acidic biological environment.

Q1.10: Can you identify two cellular zones in the pulp (the cell nuclei are stained purple)?

A: Subjacent to the pre-dentine zone is the odontoblast layer with vertically oriented cells. Beneath this layer is the sub-odontoblastic cell-rich layer.

Q1.11: How many other carious lesions can you detect?

A: Distal/mesial (d/m) UR6, d/m UR5, m LR7, d/m LR6, d/m LR5, not including the grossly broken down UR4!

Q1.12: Can you identify five histological zones in the H&E section in Figure 1.18 from top to bottom?

A: Sound dentine, reactionary dentine, pre-dentine, odontoblast layer, and the relatively undifferentiated sub-odontoblastic cell-rich layer.

Q1.13: What might have been the presenting dental complaints for the patient in Figure 1.20?

A: Pain, difficulty chewing, sharp fractured teeth/fillings against the tongue or cheeks, not being able to bite properly, poor appearance, difficulty in brushing the teeth due to sensitivity, and tooth fractures.

Q1.14: Can you detect any abnormal clinical findings from Figure 1.21 (clue—check the mucosae)?

A: Difficult, but did you notice the mucosal swelling level with the muco-gingival junction adjacent to the UL3?

Q1.15: What other findings are evident from the USO radiograph?

A: The near complete obliteration of the pulp chamber and root canal spaces in the UL1.

2

Clinical detection: 'information gathering'

Chapter contents

2.1 Introduction

The oral healthcare team (dentist, nurse, hygienist/therapist/oral health educator, laboratory technician, receptionist, practice manager), led by the principal dental practitioner, should all be involved in the decision-making processes and dental management of the patient, as part of the minimum intervention philosophy of oral/dental healthcare (see Figure 1.1 in Chapter 1). This care rationale is patient-centred, engaging with the patient to encourage them to take responsibility for their own oral health. The role of the oral healthcare team is to provide advice and guidance to help the patient to maintain oral health, as well as providing operative treatment to repair damaged hard and soft tissues. Sometimes the dentist will refer difficult cases to a specialist dentist for their opinion as to what the diagnosis and care plan should be.

To manage patients successfully, there are five stages that must be followed (see Figure 2.1):

1. Detecting clinical problems and their aetiology (see Chapter 2):
   - This involves detective work to help to gather clinically relevant and useful information, primarily using the skills of verbal history taking, oral examination, and relevant special investigations.

2. Diagnosis and risk assessment (see Chapter 3):
   - The art of interpretation of signs and symptoms/results from investigations to conclude with identifying the cause of the problem and the potential the individual patient has of developing further disease in the future or responding to treatment. Both aspects are critical to planning the overall care of the patient.

3. Prognosis (see Chapter 3):
   - The art of forecasting the course of a disease or problem, whether treated or not.

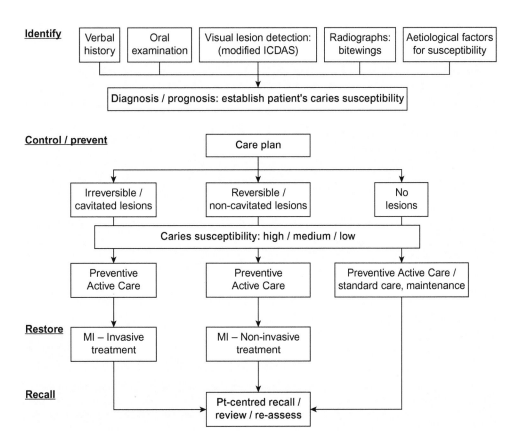

Figure 2.1 Minimum intervention patient care flowchart showing how the patient management stages of *identify* (see Chapter 2), *control and prevent* (see Chapter 4), *restore* (see Chapters 5, 6, 7, and 8), and *review/ monitor/recall* (see Chapter 9) link to one another (see also Figure 1.1 in Chapter 1). Note how the patient-centred care plan focuses on caries risk/susceptibility. The medium risk grade has been shaded to signify that at a practical patient contact level, most can be managed as either high or low risk. The key factor is that the patient's risk and susceptibility are monitored over time. Tooth wear and other conditions will be considered later in this chapter. (Reproduced from A Banerjee and S Domejean. *Primary Dental Journal, 2, 3,* pp. 30–37. © 2013, with permission from the Royal College of Surgeons.)

4. Formulation of an individualized patient care plan (see Chapters 3 and 4):

   - This must be underpinned by the non-invasive control of disease and lesion prevention, following the principles of minimum intervention oral care.
   - The care plan will also include itemized, costed, minimally invasive operative treatments when required.

5. Recall/re-assess/review (see Chapter 9):

   - Reviewing the outcomes of any care provided, re-assessing the patient's response to evaluate whether knowledge/behavioural adaptations and adherence have helped to control and/or prevent disease reoccurrence, and developing adaptive recall strategies/intervals that are patient-centred, rather than generic and guideline-driven.

2.2 Detection/identification: 'information gathering'

This aspect of patient management involves gathering the relevant information based on which sound clinical judgements can be made as to the best course of treatment for the individual patient. Clinical detection works on two levels:

- detecting the immediate clinical problem (i.e. trauma or the physical manifestation of the disease process, such as carious lesions, toothwear (TW) lesions)
- detecting and understanding the complex interplay of aetiological factors that have *caused* the problem for that particular patient over time.

It is critical that detailed notes are made for all stages of the patient management pathway, documented at every visit. This can be done using electronic patient recording systems or handwritten notes. Each patient will have their own notes with their name, date of birth, address, contact details, and occupation listed. It is essential to check that the correct notes have been called up for the attending patient, and for each visit the date and time of appointment must be noted initially.

2.3 Taking a verbal history

The art of verbal history taking (anamnesis) is the first and most important way of obtaining information about any problems the patient may present with, and also their aetiology. The answers to a series of carefully planned questions will help to shed light on the nature and severity of the problem(s) presented. A generic structured 'interview' with the clinical relevance of each question is presented in Table 2.1. Of course this is not the only format of questioning that can be used, and with experience it should be adjusted to the specific needs and conditions of the patient, and modified to assess aetiological factors of the presenting conditions (see later).

Table 2.1 Structured verbal history ordered to ask relevant questions to help unearth the clues for a diagnosis of the presenting problem and the formulation of an individualized care plan

Structuring the verbal history	Comments
Patient complains of . . . (C/O)	Document, in the patient's own words, the presenting symptom(s)/problem(s)
History of presenting complaint(s) (HPC)	*Commencement*: when did it/they start? *Location*: ask the patient to describe or ask them to point/outline the area with one finger *Type*: description of symptoms. Avoid putting words in the patient's mouth *Incidence*: how long ago did the episodes start? *Duration*: for how long do they persist? Frequency? Are they getting better, staying the same, or deteriorating? *Initiating/relieving factors*: does anything make the symptoms worse or better? **Answers to the above will often provide the clues to help direct the clinician to the correct diagnosis**
Past dental history (PDH)	What previous dental treatment has the patient experienced (orthodontics/extractions/periodontal treatment/fillings, etc.)? How regularly do they visit the dentist? What previous preventive advice have they received/do they follow? **Answers to the above will help to create a picture of the attitude/motivation of the patient towards dentistry and their own oral health, without asking them directly about these issues**

Medical history (MH)	Most oral healthcare teams use a formatted checklist, which should include information about:
	• cardiac problems/disease/rheumatic fever/blood pressure
	• respiratory disease/asthma/shortness of breath
	• diabetes/epilepsy/jaundice /hepatitis history
	• current/recent past medications
	• allergies
	• bleeding/haemorrhage/clotting defects
	• other illnesses/operations/hospital admissions
	• pregnancy
	• HIV/AIDS/communicable disease risk
	Information relevant regarding drug interactions with local anaesthetic, and allergies to latex/resins/ dental materials. Bleeding problems/anticoagulant therapies relevant for periodontal surgery, root planing, and extractions. Check medication in the *Dental Formulary* or equivalent. Medications that cause dry mouth, gingival overgrowth, or vomiting (emesis) should be noted
Social history (SH)	Occupation/family members/availability for appointments
	Relevant when considering appointment logistics to deliver the care plan for the individual
Habits	Oral hygiene (OH—procedures, frequency), use of fluoride, diet (amount/frequency of sugar intake, balanced diet, erosive potential for tooth wear), smoking, alcohol intake, parafunctional habits (bruxism (teeth grinding), clenching)
	Relevant when planning care and giving preventive advice. What the patient says might be checked/ verified during the oral examination to follow. Helps to ascertain the possible aetiology of the problem

2.4 Physical examination

Once the verbal history has been taken, a physical examination follows, which is divided into a general and oral examination.

2.4.1 General examination

This will commence as the clinician interviews the patient. The demeanour of the individual, facial/ocular asymmetries, facial nerve palsies, pallor, tremors, or mental/physical disabilities can be noted and followed up if relevant to the dental care required.

2.4.2 Oral examination

See Table 2.2. An error commonly made by inexperienced clinicians is to dive into an oral examination and direct all attention immediately to the teeth. It is better to have a system that encompasses all aspects of oral health, including the mucosal soft tissues and periodontal tissues, as well as teeth and prostheses. When examining the oral mucosae, learn a system which ensures that all aspects of the oral cavity are included, i.e. anterior to posterior (lips to tonsils), posterior to anterior, or clockwise/anticlockwise around the oral cavity. Once learned and practised, this is never forgotten, even during the stress of clinical examinations! Ensure that adequate time has been set aside for the examination, along with suitable dental instrumentation and lighting (see Chapter 5). Clinical digital photography can often assist in the documentation of any notable findings during the examination, but appropriate informed and written consent must be obtained prior to any images being captured and stored securely. Data to be recorded along with the image(s) must include patient details, the date of capture of the image(s), the clinical findings, and, where appropriate, a scale to help the viewer to assess the size of any lesion imaged. The camera settings and ambient lighting should also be noted in case comparative images are taken at a later date, to enable standardization between them. The assisting member of staff should be trained to document accurately and faithfully all of the information gathered during this part of the examination. However, the practising clinician still has ultimate responsibility for checking any records taken during the examination.

The examination of the oral cavity must also include an assessment of the quantity and quality of the patient's saliva. As has been previously mentioned, saliva plays a critical role in the control of dental disease risk, especially caries and erosion (see Section 2.5.4).

2.4.3 Dental charting

When examining the dentition, there are certain features that the dentist must relay to their assistant to record accurately in a dental chart (see Figure 2.2). This chart is interpreted as though the dentist is looking

Table 2.2 Steps involved in a comprehensive clinical oral examination. Note that a full examination should not be rushed, and careful recording of findings is essential both clinically and dento-legally

Examination site		Comments
Extra-oral		Facial swellings/asymmetries, lips—form and seal, facial and neck lymph nodes, TMJ—crepitus, clicking (uni-bilateral), mandibular movement (opening gape, deviations, lateral/protrusive excursions) **Operator stands behind the patient for the TMJ/LN exam—remember to notify the patient prior to starting!**
Intra-oral	Mucosae	All internal buccal, labial, alveolar mucosae, including vermilion border of lips, tongue (dorsum, lateral borders, and ventral surfaces), retromolar areas, hard and soft palate, and floor of mouth. Palpation of the pterygoid muscles **Checking for white or erythematous patches/plaques indicative of trauma, lichenoid reactions, or neoplastic change—referral to an oral medicine specialist might be appropriate. Tenderness in the pterygoid muscles—sign of TMD? Dry mucosae and frothy saliva are indicative of dry mouth (see Section 2.5.4)**
	Periodontium	Marginal gingivae (colour, contour, consistency), gingivitis (BPE score), recession, loss of attachment, probing depths, mobility, presence of supra-/subgingival calculus, plaque indices **Relevant to assess periodontal status, which will affect the overall restorative status of the mouth and of the individual tooth**
	Teeth	Missing teeth, mobility, restoration status, caries, tooth wear (site, enamel ± dentine), malpositioning (tilting, rotation, overeruption/submerged)
	Prostheses	Crowns, removable dentures, fixed bridges, implant-retained crown and bridge work, orthodontic appliances (fixed and removable) **Relevant regarding oral hygiene procedures, plaque-retentive margins, aesthetics, and status of abutment teeth**
	Occlusion	Angle's classification (Class I, II, and III), incisor relationship (Class I, II division 1/2, and Class III). Intercuspal position (ICP), retruded contact position (RCP), protrusive, retrusive, lateral excursive movements—working and non-working side contacts. Skeletal discrepancies **Relevant to the restoration of individual/groups of teeth to conform to the existing occlusal harmony or to assess changes in a reorganized approach in more complex care plans (see Chapter 5)**
	Saliva (see Table 2.5)	*Quality:* normal, frothy, viscous. *Quantity:* normal, reduced output, buccal mucosae/tongue sticks to mirror head, limited/no pooling in floor of mouth, shiny mucosae lobulated/fissured tongue, altered gingival architecture, glassy appearance of oral mucosa, cervical caries, food debris present **Relevant regarding the protective effects of saliva for teeth and the oral mucosae. Low saliva output/ poor quality increases patient risk of caries and oral infections**

TMJ, temporomandibular joint; LN, lymph node; TMD, temporomandibular dysfunction; BPE, Basic Periodontal Examination.

at the patient face to face, and the notation is communicated from the patient's perspective.

1. Which tooth, side, position (e.g. 'upper left 6' or 'upper left first permanent molar', rotated/tilted/space-closed).

2. Presence of existing restoration(s)—location (mesio-occlusal, buccal, cervical, etc.) and type of material (amalgam, tooth-coloured, gold, ceramic, etc.).

3. Status of existing restorations—sound, or deficient margins/ fractured/missing.

4. Presence of carious lesion(s)—location, mICDAS classification (see Table 2.3), lesion activity.

5. Presence of tooth wear—location (buccal, occlusal, incisal) and extent (in enamel or dentine, exposing pulp, BEWE score) (see Table 2.7).

6. Presence of other abnormalities (e.g. fluorosis, hypoplastic enamel, cracks).

With practice, this can be done with a series of abbreviated responses, and good teamwork with the nurse/assistant can expedite

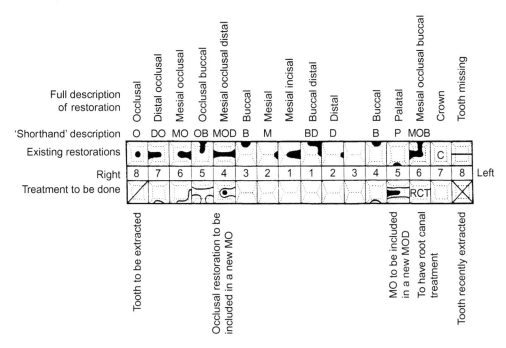

Figure 2.2 Conventions for recording restorations, lesions/teeth requiring restoration, teeth to be extracted, and other conditions on a dental chart.

Q2.1: Can you spot an error in the charting in Figure 2.2?

this process. Of course, if points 2–6 in this list do not apply after careful examination, a summary of 'sound' will usually suffice and a dot is placed on the relevant tooth in the chart. It is important to check all five surfaces of each tooth either with direct vision or using the dental mirror and good lighting of a clean tooth. It might be necessary in some patients, before the visual examination (but after checking any relevant medical history), to clean the dentition with a periodontal hand/ultrasonic scaler in order to remove supragingival plaque and calculus deposits that might be obscuring the clear view of the tooth surfaces beneath.

2.4.4 Tooth notation

In the UK, the most commonly used notations are the Palmer system and a two-letter coding system. Both are shown in Figure 2.3, dividing the mouth into four quadrants with the teeth in each numbered from 1 to 8 from central incisors to third molars.

A drawback of the Palmer notation is that this can be difficult to input into electronic notes (although current software packages are accommodating this system).

Two numerical notation systems exist—the FDI (Federation Dentaire Internationale, favoured in mainland Europe; see Figure 2.4) and the Universal system (favoured in the USA; see Figure 2.5). Users tend to credit these systems for crossing language boundaries, but confusion can easily occur with these solely numerical notations—for example, FDI 16 (see Figure 2.4) represents UR6 (upper right first permanent

molar, 6|), whereas Universal 16 (see Figure 2.5) represents UL8 (upper left third permanent molar, |8).

UR	8 7 6 5 4 3 2 1	1 2 3 4 5 6 7 8	UL
LR	8 7 6 5 4 3 2 1	1 2 3 4 5 6 7 8	LL

Figure 2.3 The Palmer and two-letter coding systems (UR, upper right; UL, upper left; LR, lower right; LL, lower left) communicated as though the dentist is looking directly at the patient. In both systems the deciduous dentition is labelled a–e from the midline.

UR	18 17 16 15 14 13 12 11	21 22 23 24 25 26 27 28	UL
LR	48 47 46 45 44 43 42 41	31 32 33 34 35 36 37 38	LL

Figure 2.4 The FDI tooth notation system with the teeth in each quadrant prefixed by a number from 1 to 4.

UR	1 2 3 4 5 6 7 8	9 10 11 12 13 14 15 16	UL
LR	32 31 30 29 28 27 26 25	24 23 22 21 20 19 18 17	LL

Figure 2.5 The Universal tooth notation system, with each individual tooth being allocated a number from 1 to 32 in the permanent dentition.

Table 2.3 A modified ICDAS (mICDAS) carious lesion scoring system (0–4), linking the clinical appearance with the equivalent underlying lesion histology. Images show teeth sectioned longitudinally through occlusal lesions, as representative clinical examples of each mICDAS score. This clinical scoring system is useful for inclusion in the patient's notes, for monitoring, and for dento-legal purposes.

0 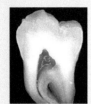 Clinical appearance: No or slight change in enamel translucency after prolonged air drying (> 5 s)
Underlying histology: No enamel demineralization or a narrow surface zone of opacity

1 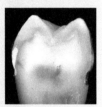 Clinical appearance: Opacity or discoloration from the enamel (white spot lesion) hardly visible on a wet surface, but distinctly visible after air drying. No cavitation on occlusal/smooth surfaces
Underlying histology: Enamel demineralization limited to outer 50%

2 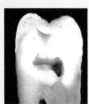 Clinical appearance: Enamel opacity (white spot lesion) or greyish discoloration distinctly visible without the need for air drying. No clinical cavitation detectable
Underlying histology: Demineralization involving inner 50% of enamel through to the outer third of dentine

3  Clinical appearance: Localized enamel breakdown in opaque or discolored enamel, ± greyish discoloration/shadowing from underlying dentine
Underlying histology: Demineralization involving the middle to inner third of dentine

4 Clinical appearance: Gross cavitation in opaque or discoloured enamel exposing the underlying stained dentine
Underlying histology: Demineralization involving the inner third of dentine towards pulp

2.5 Caries detection

Visual detection of carious lesions in enamel and dentine relies on the following operator-controlled factors:

- Using 'sharp' eyes and the recommended use of magnification in the form of dental loupes (see Chapter 5).
- Using good illumination from the overhead dental chair light or a more focused light from an LED headlight, usually coupled with the use of magnification loupes.
- Having clean tooth surfaces to examine both wet and dry (using a 3-1 air/water syringe; see Figure 2.6(a) and (b)). If surface debris (plaque/calculus) is present, this may have to be removed prior to any dental examination taking place (see Figure 2.6 (a) and (b) and Figure 1.2 (b) and (c)).

- Using rounded/ball-ended dental explorers—the use of sharp dental probes is contraindicated for carious lesion detection as they can, with injudicious use, cause cavitation in a previously non-cavitated lesion (see Figure 2.7).
- Separating teeth may be beneficial to assess the proximal surfaces of adjacent teeth visually, ideally with magnification. Wedges or orthodontic separators can be placed interproximally for a few minutes prior to the examination of the field, to gently displace the gingiva apically and part the teeth slightly through movement within their periodontal ligament spaces. In this way, incipient or cavitated lesions may become more evident.
- Sufficient time allocated for the examination of all tooth surfaces as well as the soft tissues and periodontium.

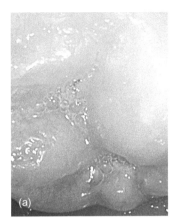
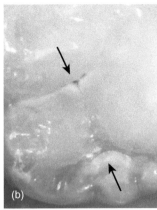

Figure 2.6 **(a)** A maxillary molar that is apparently caries-free with saliva obscuring the occlusal fissures. **(b)** When the saliva is removed with the 3-1 air/water syringe, an incipient white spot lesion becomes evident (mICDAS 1). (Courtesy of L. Mackenzie.)

Q2.2: What hand instrument (in Fig 2.7) should be used instead and for what purpose?

2.5.1 Caries detection indices

The histopathology and clinical signs of the carious lesion have been described in Chapter 1. The clinical manifestation of the caries process is the progressive lesion it creates within the dental hard tissues. A dentist must be able to link the visual clinical appearance of the lesion with the underlying histological damage that has occurred in the tooth (and possibly lesion activity status), at a particular moment in time. In this way the dentist can then diagnose problems, and decide how to manage the lesion/disease process in that individual patient through the development of a suitable care plan. In an attempt to do this, as well as for reviewing the relative success or failure of previous treatment at recall consultations and to help with dento-legal documentation, several visual indices have been described over the years. In 2004, the ICDAS (International Caries Detection and Assessment System) Foundation was convened to produce an evidence-based clinical caries assessment system to be used primarily for epidemiological and research studies, as well as in general dental practice (see QR code image 2.1).

QR code image 2.1 Scan this code with your mobile device to view the International Caries Detection and Assessment System.

www.icdas.org

A simpler, modified version is presented in Table 2.3 with clinical examples (see Figures 2.6, 2.8, 2.9, and 2.10), which permits the dentist to examine clinically the tooth surface and appreciate the underlying damage that has been caused. Then, depending on the individual's caries risk assessment, the most relevant treatment option can be chosen. This index requires that the points listed and discussed previously are implemented judiciously, and allows an objective numerical record to be made in the dental chart to permit longitudinal, dento-legally appropriate assessment of the particular lesion over time.

Alternative indices exist for classifying carious lesions. The 'caries iceberg', developed in collaboration with cariologists and epidemiologists, is an index used by many experts to study the incidence and

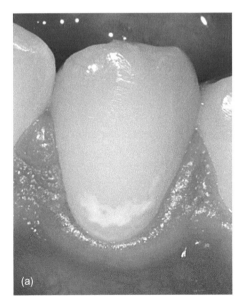
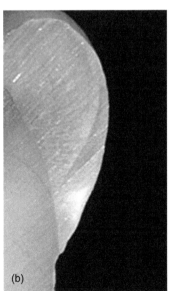
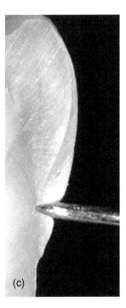
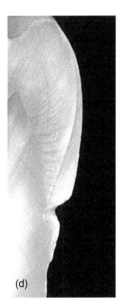

Figure 2.7 **(a)** A smooth surface incipient white spot lesion (WSL) associated with the cervical aspect of a mandibular canine. **(b)** A cross-section through an equivalent buccal cervical WSL showing the classical 'inverted cone' shape of the non-cavitated enamel lesion (see Chapter 1, Section 1.2.6). **(c)** This lesion has been probed using a sharp dental explorer resulting in **(d)** operator-induced (iatrogenic) cavitation of the lesion that should have been managed non-operatively. The use of a sharp dental probe to elicit 'sticky fissures/surfaces' is contraindicated for caries detection. (Courtesy of L. Mackenzie.)

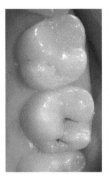
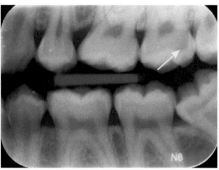

Figure 2.8 The brown, non-cavitated fissures with underlying grey discoloration on the occlusal surface of the UL7 are caused by demineralized, discoloured dentine shining through intact, wet enamel (a closed lesion, visible in dentine on the bitewing radiograph (right, yellow arrow)—mICDAS 2).

Q2.3: What treatment may be required for the tooth shown in Figure 2.8?

prevalence of the disease in different populations. This permits the development of strategies to manage caries at a population level as well as at a patient level. The 'iceberg' can be seen in Figure 2.11—clinically detectable lesions are divided into four groups, D1–D4, depending on the depth of tissue invasion and the degree of cavitation. Note that careful selection of caries detection thresholds is required, otherwise this index may lead to threshold bias when interpreting data for caries prevalence in a population. For example, if D3 detection threshold (dentine lesions, cavitated or not, i.e. open or closed) is selected to establish the presence/absence of caries, patients with early-stage lesions within enamel, cavitated or not, will not be included in the final data, thus incorrectly reducing the caries prevalence for that particular population.

2.5.2 Susceptible surfaces

Carious lesions occur on tooth surfaces that have accumulated plaque biofilm which has been allowed to stagnate for a prolonged period of time. During the clinical examination, it would be prudent to examine these areas with particular care, for early signs of lesions:

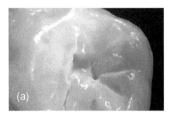
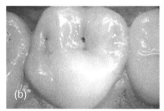

Figure 2.9 (a), (b) A small cavity is just detectable within the whitish opacity/brown discoloration on the occlusal surfaces of these molars, appearing as a widened fissure and a cavitated pit, respectively. They can easily be missed clinically unless the surfaces are clean and vision aided by the use of magnification. Histologically, both lesions were well into dentine, visible on radiographs—mICDAS 3.

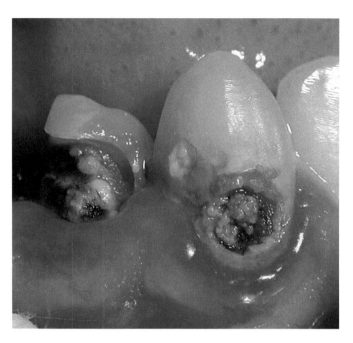

Figure 2.10 Grossly cavitated buccal carious lesions on LR3 and LR4, with quantities of stagnant dense plaque deposited on the exposed dentine—mICDAS 4.

- The depths of pits and fissures on posterior occlusal surfaces (which cannot be cleaned effectively with a toothbrush). These areas on newly erupting, partially erupted, or submerged molars are particularly susceptible to carious attack.

- Proximal surfaces (mesial and distal) *cervical* to contact points of adjacent teeth (where patients may not floss regularly, or at all). The surfaces of particularly imbricated (crowded) teeth can be more susceptible due to the lack of access to oral hygiene aids.

- Smooth surfaces adjacent to the gingival margin (again where patients often miss with their toothbrush).

- The ledged/overhanging/deficient margins of existing restorations (a plaque trap often inaccessible to a toothbrush/floss).

Of course, these are not the only sites on which carious lesions occur. The site and distribution of lesions in a patient's mouth might give an indication of underlying aetiological factors. For example, patients with xerostomia (dry mouth) due to salivary gland disease or damage (e.g. from radiotherapy when treating head and neck cancers) can develop lesions on the incisal surfaces of anterior teeth and lesions that circumvent the neck of the crown at the gingival margin. Patients with eating disorders may have lesions on the lingual-cervical aspect of the mandibular teeth (see Figure 2.12).

2.5.3 Special investigations

To aid the process of clinical information gathering, other investigations may be requested, the results of which must be interpreted clinically to help to verify or make the final diagnosis of the problem and possibly its aetiology. Investigations have a cost implication for the patient or the health service provider and, depending on the test, may be invasive or even potentially harmful in nature. It is imperative that information

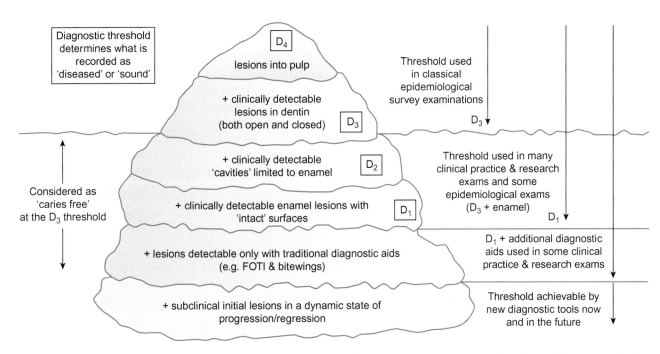

Diagnostic threshold determines what is recorded as 'diseased' or 'sound'

D₄
lesions into pulp

+ clinically detectable lesions in dentin (both open and closed) D₃

+ clinically detectable 'cavities' limited to enamel D₂

+ clinically detectable enamel lesions with 'intact' surfaces D₁

+ lesions detectable only with traditional diagnostic aids (e.g. FOTI & bitewings)

+ subclinical initial lesions in a dynamic state of progression/regression

Threshold used in classical epidemiological survey examinations D₃

Threshold used in many clinical practice & research exams and some epidemiological exams (D₃ + enamel) D₁

D₁ + additional diagnostic aids used in some clinical practice & research exams

Threshold achievable by new diagnostic tools now and in the future

Considered as 'caries free' at the D₃ threshold

Figure 2.11 The 'caries iceberg' classifying clinically detectable lesions with regard to their level of tissue invasion and degree of cavitation. (Reproduced from NB Pitts 'Diagnostic tools and measurements – impact on appropriate care.' *Community Dentistry and Oral Epidemiology*, 25, pp. 24–35. © 1997, with permission from John Wiley & Sons Ltd.)

gathered using multiple special investigations is not interpreted individually, but in conjunction with all of the other methods described in this chapter to help to formulate the diagnosis for the patient. All investigations are prone to false-positive and false-negative outcomes. Analysing the relative proportions of these outcomes, statistical measures of *sensitivity* (the measure of how effective an investigation is at detecting true disease), *specificity* (the measure of how effective an investigation is at detecting true health), and the *positive predictive value (ppv—that is, true positives divided by the sum of true and false positives)* can be developed, which are useful in assessing the investigation's value in providing

a clinically relevant diagnostic yield. For caries detection, these include intra-oral radiographs, pulp vitality (sensibility) and percussion tests.

Radiographs

Horizontal bitewing radiographs should be used to aid lesion detection on proximal surfaces of posterior teeth, especially when adjacent teeth are present and direct vision is not possible. A film holder and beam-aiming device should be used routinely in order to obtain the optimal angulation of the beam perpendicular to the contact points and to allow reproducibility of films when monitoring lesions over a period of time (see Figure 2.13).

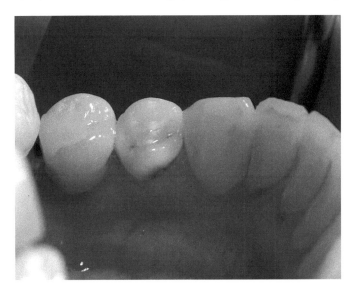

Figure 2.12 A patient with an eating disorder, anorexia nervosa, with carious cavitated lesions on the lingual aspects of LL124 (mICDAS 2,3).

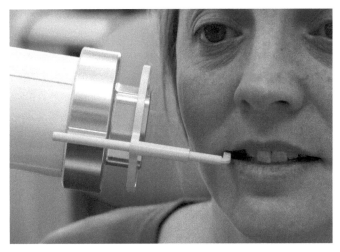

Figure 2.13 Right bitewing radiograph being taken with film holder and beam-aiming device (yellow arm) enabling optimal alignment of the radiographic beam at right angles to the teeth and intra-oral film.

Incipient occlusal lesions are difficult to detect, and only later-stage occlusal lesions are clearly visible on these radiographs. Periapical radiographs may be used to assess the depth of proximal lesions in anterior teeth. Dental panoramic tomogram radiographs (sometimes also called DPTs, OPTs, or OPGs) should not be used routinely for caries detection, due to their limited resolution, potential for distortion, and increased radiation dose by comparison with small intra-oral films. The radiographic appearance of caries (radiolucency in enamel or dentine) is often described as being up to 6 months behind the actual histological spread of the lesion in the tooth. Therefore a lesion radiographically encased within enamel may have actually spread histologically across the enamel–dentine junction (EDJ) into the outer third of dentine. This is because intra-oral radiography, at the clinical radiation dose used conventionally, has only sufficient sensitivity to detect relatively gross changes in mineral density. As the beam passes through quantities of potentially sound, highly mineralized tissues in a tooth, zones of early demineralization will be masked and therefore undetectable on the film/plate/detector. Thus conventional radiography can detect only the demineralization in more extensive enamel lesions and the caries-infected dentine of the deeper lesion (see Chapter 1, Section 1.2.6). Remember that radiographs are two-dimensional representations of the change in radio-density of a three-dimensional object, taken as a snapshot in time. Studies have shown that once a carious lesion has progressed radiographically just into the middle third of dentine, the enamel is likely to be grossly demineralized and cavitated.

Table 2.4 shows how the mICDAS scores for the visual and histological lesion appearance correlate with the radiographic appearance/depth of enamel and dentine lesions. Examples of lesions detected from bitewing radiographs of a high caries risk patient are shown in Figure 2.14 (a) and (b). Once experience has been gained in interpreting radiographs, other clues can often be found to help with the diagnosis and potential activity status of the lesion(s). These might include the outline of the pulp horns—often tertiary dentine has been laid down in response to the active disease process, and this can be observed by the relative shrinkage of the radiolucent pulp horn subjacent to the spreading lesion. In addition, the 'moth-eaten' appearance of the advancing edge of the radiolucency is a clue that, at the time when the film was taken, the

lesion was in a state of relative activity causing demineralization. If the dentine–pulp complex has had a chance to lay down extra mineral to 'wall off' the lesion (a more defined radio-opaque boundary), this implies a relative tipping of the metabolic balance towards inactivity and healing.

It is imperative that the dentist does not immediately start to treat operatively a radiolucency on a radiograph alone, without considering all of the other clinical findings, signs, and symptoms. A diagnosis must be made on the basis of all the information that has been discussed in this section, prior to any operative intervention. Radiographic radiolucencies/radio-opacities in teeth may be caused by:

- pathology (e.g. caries, internal resorption, pulp calcifications)
- natural anatomy (e.g. pulp chamber morphology, rotations/malpositioning of teeth, anatomical superimposition, canine fossae in first premolars)
- artefact (e.g. cervical burnout in the proximal region of the tooth close to the alveolar crest mimicking proximal caries; see Figure 2.14 c)
- restorative process (e.g. radiolucent/opaque restorative materials; see Figure 2.14 c, d, and e).

Figures 2.14c, d, and e show examples of potential conundrums that a clinician may encounter when interpreting the causes of differing radio-densities in bitewing or other radiographs. An 'obvious' initial diagnosis of active caries made from detecting the well-demarcated radiolucency in Figure 2.14c does not correlate with the clinical findings for the same tooth (see Figure 2.14 d). So what is the cause? (See answer to Self-Assessment Question 2.5.) The diffuse radiolucency just subjacent to the restoration in the maxillary molar in Figure 2.14e poses an interesting dilemma. This laminate restoration was placed after minimally invasive caries excavation (see Chapter 5, Section 5.9) and the digital radiograph was taken at the 1-year recall consultation. Such an appearance might be caused by any of the following:

- residual, inactive caries retained during the minimally invasive caries excavation procedure
- active caries due to microleakage at the proximal restoration margin
- the presence of a radiolucent pulp protection material (see Chapter 5, Section 5.11)
- the possible effect on dentine of the restorative adhesive process (e.g. adhesive procedure, dental adhesive; see Figure 7.16f in Chapter 7).

In such cases, it is imperative to examine the tooth/restoration carefully and to check signs and symptoms with the patient. Findings from other special investigations may be required (see later). Collectively, this information will help the dentist to ascertain the cause of the radiographic finding and thus to decide whether it is necessary to manage the situation operatively or preventively. Examination of the patient notes and any previous radiographs and their radiographic reporting will also be useful in this context.

Just taking and filing radiographs in the patient's notes is not acceptable. It is essential that a comprehensive report of all the radiographic findings is documented in the patient's notes for long-term scrutiny, for monitoring, and for dento-legal reasons.

Table 2.4 The association between the radiographic lesion depth (E1–D3) and equivalent mICDAS scores

Enamel Lesion		mICDAS
E1	Outer half of enamel	0, 1
E2	Inner half of enamel	1

Dentine Lesion		mICDAS
D1	Outer third of dentine	2
D2	Middle third of dentine	3
D3	Inner third of dentine	4

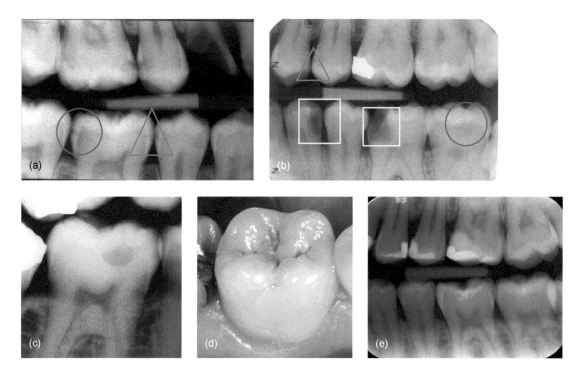

Figure 2.14 **(a)** Right and **(b)** left bitewing radiographs from two different patients, both with high caries experience, showing carious lesions within enamel and outer third dentine (E2–D1, blue triangle), approaching middle third of dentine (D2, red circle), and very close to the pulp (D3, yellow square). Note that other lesions can be detected on these films. **(c)** Well-defined radiolucency in the occlusal aspect of the mandibular molar, as well as radiolucencies present at the cervical aspects both mesially and distally. **(d)** Clinical image of the mandibular molar whose radiograph is shown in (c). **(e)** Left bitewing radiograph focusing on the maxillary and mandibular first molars. Note the radio-opacity associated with the occlusal aspect of the mandibular molar. The maxillary first molar has received a proximo-occlusal restoration to treat a large carious lesion. Note the differences in radio-density between the different restorative materials, enamel and dentine. Note also the diffuse radiolucency between the deepest aspect of the restoration and the pulp chamber (see text for explanation). (Figures 2.14 (c) and (d) courtesy of L Mackenzie.)

Q2.4: Can you find more lesions in Figure 2.14 (a) and (b) and classify them radiographically? Can you comment on the radiographic changes of the pulp chambers in those teeth?

Q2.5: What is the cause of the radiolucencies in Figure 2.14(c)? (Clue—look carefully at (d) for the answer!)

Q2.6:

i Can you guess which materials have been used to restore the cavity in the maxillary molar in Figure 2.14(e)?

ii What other information would you need before deciding to operatively intervene or not, to manage the diffuse radiolucency subjacent to the restoration?

iii What might be the cause of the radio-opacity in the mandibular molar?

Pulp vitality (sensibility) tests

Technically, the term 'vitality' implies the status of pulpal blood flow. This can be measured using laser Doppler flowmetry, which has been mainly applied for research purposes. Clinical signs of a non-vital, necrotic pulp may include the following:

- Discoloration and darkening of the tooth due to the breakdown products of haemoglobin in the pulp chamber. Greying and reduced translucency might also be noticed. These changes may be difficult to detect if the tooth is heavily restored or has an extracoronal restoration covering it.

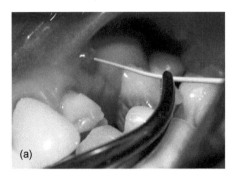
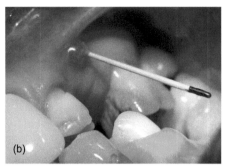
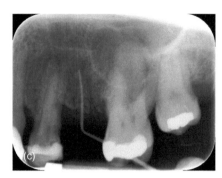

Figure 2.15 **(a)** A soft, non-tender swelling on the dentoalveolar mucosa distally adjacent to the periapical region of the broken-down UL4, a chronic sinus, into which a sterile gutta-percha point has been carefully inserted **(b)** and radiograph showing the exact location of the 'abscess' **(c)**. The UL6 is vital with no symptoms.

- Over time, a necrotic pulp may give rise to a sinus, tracking from the periapical tissues to the mucosal surface usually adjacent to the apex of the tooth in question. A gutta-percha point inserted gently into the endodontic sinus and then radiographed will show the direction of the sinus track and ultimately the periapical origin of the infection (see Figure 2.15).

The status of pulp innervation (sensibility) can be assessed to ascertain the effect of the caries process on the pulp:

- *Temperature*: heat from warm gutta-percha sticks (rare) or, more commonly, cold from cotton wool pledgets soaked in ethyl chloride or ice sticks may be used to ascertain the status of pulpal innervation. Tooth surfaces to be assessed must be dry and clear of surface debris (plaque/calculus; see Figure 2.16). Check equivalent teeth on the contralateral side to the tooth in question and then the adjacent teeth (acting as an internal control), ensuring that the cotton wool/ice stick/gutta-percha is placed on a clean, dry, sound tooth surface. Ask the patient to raise a hand when they feel a sensation in the tooth being tested. Vital teeth tend to respond quickly, whereas false-positive readings respond more slowly (conduction through dentine/metallic restoration into the periodontal membrane).
- *Electrical*: a monopolar electric pulp test unit passes a small current (direct or alternating) through the patient and the tooth with which it is in contact. The patient's hand must be in contact with the metal handle of the handpiece to complete the circuit with some commercial systems. The probe is placed on a clean, sound tooth surface (contralateral and adjacent equivalents are tested first as an internal patient control) using an electrolytic coupling agent on the tooth surface to ensure completion of the circuit (usually a small amount of prophylaxis paste; see Figure 2.17). The current is increased gradually by the dentist until the patient feels a tingling sensation in the tooth. At this point they are instructed to let go of the handpiece and the circuit is broken. The numerical value can be recorded and is useful for monitoring purposes for a particular tooth, but is not equivocal as the readings can vary from the same patient. False-positive responses may be elicited through stimulation of nerve fibres in the periodontium, and in posterior multi-rooted teeth a mixture of vital and non-vital pulp tissue may confound the interpretation of the reading.
- *Cutting a test cavity without local anaesthesia*: a rarely used, invasive last resort that checks the innervation of the dentine–pulp complex by drilling into potentially vital dentine. If the patient feels pain then at least partial innervation of the pulp remains.

It is important to note in the cases just described that a positive response from the pulp does not necessarily mean all is well. There is no clinical way of knowing if there is partial necrosis or denervation in a dental pulp, and multi-rooted teeth can present with partially diseased

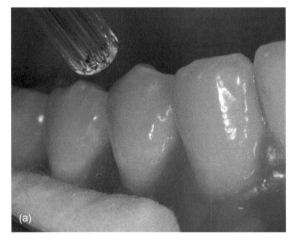
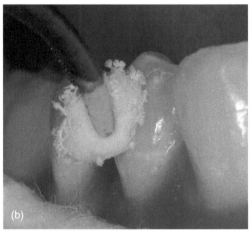

Figure 2.16 **(a)** Pulp sensibility testing of cleaned and air-dried LR4 using cold ethyl chloride-soaked cotton wool pledget. **(b)** Avoid restorations and the gingival margin, as false-positive readings may ensue.

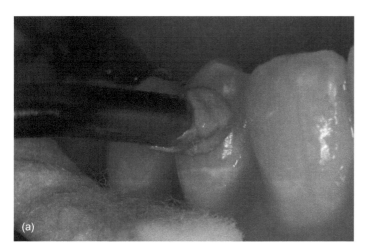

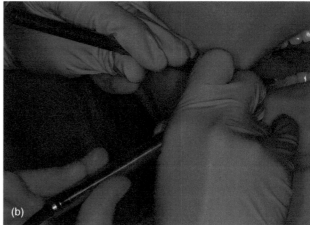

Figure 2.17 **(a)** Probe of the electric pulp tester placed on clean dry tooth surface, coupled with prophylaxis paste. **(b)** Note the patient's fingers (ungloved) touching the probe handle, so completing the electrical circuit. They should let go to break the circuit when a sensation is felt in the tooth.

pulpal tissue. Indeed, the clinical assessment of histological pulp status is not a pure, objective science, and requires interpretation of all clinical findings associated with the tooth in question.

Percussion tests

Percussion tests (gently tapping the crown axially and then obliquely with a probe or mirror handle) assess the physical condition of the periapical tissues and periodontal membrane, but not of the pulp directly. If periapical periodontitis is present, the piston-like effect of the tooth being pushed into the inflamed periapical tissues will elicit acute tenderness. The inflammation in the periodontal tissues might be caused by the toxins from a non-vital pulp.

2.5.4 Lesion activity: risk assessment

Once a carious lesion has been detected, it is important to ascertain whether it is *active* (a state where the disease process is more likely to be progressing or regressing) or *inactive* (a state where it is less likely

to be in transition, or is even arrested), so that the correct care plan can be implemented. This is difficult to define and measure objectively intra-orally at present, but certain clues can be gleaned from the following:

- *Colour and surface texture of a cavitated lesion*: an arrested lesion is often darker in colour, and the exposed dentine has a flint-like, hard, shiny outer surface when probed (see Chapter 1, Table 1.1).

- *Presence of gingival bleeding on the same tooth*: the presence of a gingival inflammatory reaction implies poor oral hygiene in that area, which will increase the risk of plaque accumulation, so making it more likely that the lesion will be in an active state of metabolic transition.

- *Presence of plaque*: if a thick biofilm overlies the lesion, it can reasonably be assumed that it is in a state of activity, as it is the presence of the plaque biofilm that is critical to the development of the carious lesion (see Figure 2.18a). If plaque can be found on non-retentive sites, again this implies poor oral hygiene measures and therefore an increased risk of caries incidence.

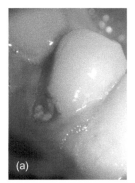

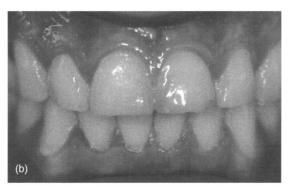

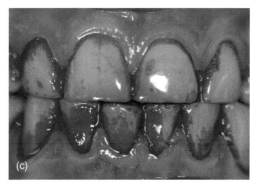

Figure 2.18 **(a)** Plaque biofilm on the surface of a buccal cervical carious lesion, indicating its potential activity. **(b)** Anterior view of dentition with a 36-hour accumulation of plaque. **(c)** A two-tone plaque indicator applied (dark blue and pink), highlighting the differing densities of plaque accumulated on the labial and gingival margins of the same teeth as in (b).

Q2.7: How could you manage the case shown in Figure 2.18?

- *Accessibility to OH procedures*: if lesions are present in uncleansable sites (see earlier), again it is likely that the lesions will be active, as a biofilm will remain on their surfaces.

- *Use of plaque indicators* (see Figure 2.18b and c): dental manufacturers have produced two- and three-tone plaque-disclosing solutions/gels which can give the practitioner and patient an indication not only of the surfaces on which the plaque biofilm is stagnating, but also for how long, as well as the plaque density and acid levels present at the tooth surface. The bacterial population (and the cariogenicity) of the biofilm develops in a structured manner in correlation with its age—the older the plaque, the more anaerobic and acidic the conditions on the enamel surface are likely to be. These proprietary kits assess neither the direct activity of lesions nor patient susceptibility to caries from the relative quantities, age, and acidogenicity of plaque, but can usefully add to all the other information gathered from the history and examination, so helping to formulate an overall picture of the individual's susceptibility and likelihood to suffer from caries in the future. They can also be helpful as strong motivators for patients, coupled with intra-oral clinical photographs to show them the problems directly, to help to improve their own oral health with better oral hygiene procedures that can be easily demonstrated.

- *Use of saliva tests*: The absence of saliva or the presence of a reduced quality of saliva is an important aetiological factor in the increased susceptibility of patients to caries and tooth wear, and more specifically erosion. More individuals (especially the elderly) are taking multiple medications ('polypharmacy') with the synergistic negative side effect of increased dry mouth (xerostomia), leading to a prevalence of this condition, stated to be affecting approximately 20% of the UK population at present. Volumetric and flow rate analyses can be carried out using simple chairside kits to assess unstimulated and stimulated salivary flow/volume, and crude levels of *Streptococcus mutans* (an indicator of the caries process) can also be calculated. The quality of the saliva can also be documented and monitored using a clinical oral dryness index (see QR code image 2.2 and Table 2.5). If the results from volumetric/flow rate analyses indicate low salivary output and there are high levels of *Streptococcus mutans* in a sample of the patient's saliva, then, *in conjunction with the results of other clinical investigations*, the dentist may collate evidence that points to the patient having a higher caries risk, and any lesions present having an increased likelihood of being active.

QR code image 2.2 Scan this code with your mobile device to view the Challacombe Scale of Oral Dryness, with accompanying images.

www.
dentalhealth.
org/uploads/
download/
resourcefiles/
download_68_1_
The%20
Challacombe
%20Scale.pdf

Table 2.5 is a text-only version of the scale.

These assessments need to be carried out periodically over time. After initial recorded baseline investigations in patients deemed to

Table 2.5 Challacombe Scale of Oral Dryness (scan QR code image 2.2 for images). This scale provides an additive score ranging from 1 (least severe) to 10 (most severe). Each feature scores 1, and symptoms will not necessarily progress in the order shown, but the total score indicates likely patient needs. Score changes over time can be used to monitor symptom progression or regression.

Score	Clinical findings	Interpretation
1	Mirror sticks to buccal mucosa	An additive score of 1–3 indicates mild dryness. May not need treatment or management. Sugar-free chewing gum for 15 minutes, twice daily, and attention to hydration is needed. Many drugs will cause mild dryness. Routine check-up and monitoring are required
2	Mirror sticks to tongue	
3	Saliva frothy	
4	No saliva pooling in floor of mouth	An additive score of 4–6 indicates moderate dryness. Sugar-free chewing gum or simple sialogogues may be required. Needs to be investigated further if the reasons for dryness are unclear. Saliva substitutes and topical fluoride may be helpful. Monitor at regular intervals, especially for early decay and symptom change
5	Tongue shows generalized shortened papillae (mild depapillation)	
6	Altered gingival architecture (i.e. smooth)	
7	Glossy appearance of oral mucosa, especially palate	An additive score of 7–10 indicates severe dryness. Saliva substitutes and topical fluoride are usually needed. Cause of hyposalivation needs to be ascertained, and Sjögren's syndrome excluded. Refer for investigation and diagnosis. Patient then needs to be monitored for changing symptoms and signs, with possible further specialist input if condition is worsening
8	Tongue lobulated/fissured	
9	Cervical caries (more than two teeth)	
10	Debris on palate or sticking to teeth	

be at risk of caries, follow-up tests may be performed at predefined, patient-specific recall intervals. This will help to evaluate the patient's risk and susceptibility over time, and thus allow their care to be planned accordingly. Patients categorized as low risk do not necessarily need continuous testing, as this may prove expensive and provide no positive clinical benefit.

2.5.5 Diet analysis

The primary aetiological factors for dental caries, as described in Chapter 1, include a susceptible tooth surface, presence of bacteria, fermentable carbohydrates, and enough time for the combination to start demineralizing the tooth surface beneath the thickened plaque biofilm. The surfaces of the teeth can be examined for carious lesions, and the bacterial levels in plaque and saliva can be investigated (see Section 2.5.4). The other main aetiological factor that can be assessed during this detection phase of patient management is dietary intake of refined carbohydrate and sugar levels in patients exhibiting signs of high caries risk (multiple lesions (> 2) developed within the previous 2 years). This is done by asking the patient to fill out a diet analysis sheet (see Figure 2.19), usually over a period of at least 3 days, encompassing the weekend. They should

be advised to write down everything that passes between their lips in that time (including water, the numbers of spoons of sugar in tea/coffee, etc.), and to note when they brush their teeth.

No indication of the relevance of the diet analysis should be given at the first appointment, so as not to bias the patient or allow them to cheat by writing down a diet intake that they feel is an improvement on what they are actually doing! The results should then be analysed by the dentist and/or trained members of the oral healthcare team, and an appointment made to discuss them. Issues to look out for are frequency of meals, hidden sugar content (e.g. many sauces/condiments are high in sugar), medications, and drinks (additional sugar/high sugar content/erosive potential due to their high titratable acidity). It is imperative that the whole team works with the patient to *modify* their existing dietary habits. Chastising the patient and ordering them to change will have the opposite effect! Work with positive reinforcement, offering suggestions or allowing the patient to make sensible suggestions to lower their sugar intake, frequency, and duration. Remember that positive encouragement to instigate small changes over time is most likely to result in positive long-term behavioural adherence. Motivational interviewing skills are a valuable asset in helping to alter patient attitudes and adherence to advice.

	Thursday			Friday			Saturday			Sunday		
	Time	Item	Ⓢ	Time	Item	Ⓢ	Time	Item	Ⓢ	Time	Item	Ⓢ
Before breakfast	7.30	Tea*		7.0	Tea*		7.30	Tea*		7.05	Tea*	
Breakfast	8.00	2 Wheat slices 2 Crisp bread 1 Apple Coffee*		8.00	2 Wheat slices 2 Crisp bread 1 Apple Coffee*		8.30	2 Wheat slices 2 Crispbread 1 Apple Coffee*		8.05	2 Wheat slices 2 Crispbread 1 Apple Coffee*	
Morning	9.00	Polo		10.00 / 11.30	Murray mint / Tea* Biscuit		11.15	Tea*		10.00 / 12.30	Lemon Barley / Tea*	
Mid-day Meal	12.30	Meat roll Tea*		2.00	Steamed fish Parsley sauce Boiled potatoes		1.45	Sausage, onion, Boiled potatoes Ice Cream, tinned fruit		1.40	Roast lamb, potatoes, cabbage, carrots	
Afternoon	2.00 / 5.30	2 Cream crackers 1 Dairy Lea Tea* / 2 Shortbread biscuits Tea*		2.45 / 6.00	Tea* / Tea*		2.30 / 5.45	Tea* / Tea*		2.00 / 4.00	Tea* / Tea*	
Evening Meal	8.00	Chop, leeks, boiled potatoes Choc-ice Tea*		8.30	Bacon sandwich Tea*		7.30	Fried kipper bread and butter		8.15	Ham salad, bread and butter Tea*	
Evening and night	1.00	Horlicks* Biscuits		10.00 / 1.30	Peanuts / Horlicks* Biscuit		9.15 / 1.45	Chocolate / Horlicks* Biscuits		1.15	Horlicks* Biscuits	

Figure 2.19 Diet analysis sheet filled in by a middle-aged man with a high incidence of caries.

Q2.8: What stands out as the main problem regarding the sugar intake of the patient in Figure 2.19?

2.5.6 Caries detection technologies

As an adjunct to the principles and methods described previously, there are other technologies available to help the dentist to detect carious lesions. Examples of some of these are shown in Table 2.6. Many detection technologies work on four basic physical principles that affect macro/microscopic changes in mineralized dental tissues, namely optical light scattering, mineral density changes, fluorescent characteristics, and tissue porosity. It is clear from this list that the currently available caries detection devices all work by assessing levels of tissue damage that have already occurred. It is arguable that these technologies do not go far enough—perhaps the ideal detection device is one that detects changes in biochemical/metabolic activity changes which would lead to tissue damage if left unchecked (i.e. detection of lesions before they actually present).

It is important to understand how a particular technology works, in order to be able to interpret accurately the information that it is providing. An example of such an ambiguity is the DiagnoDent laser-fluorescence caries detection system. Note that in Table 2.6, this system has been placed within two categories—optical light scattering and fluorescent characteristics—as clinical research has shown that the unit is affected by both properties to a varying degree. Therefore the clinical interpretation of results—that is, whether to cut a cavity or not—must be undertaken with caution in the clinical environment, again in conjunction with all of the other information gathered for the particular patient. Remember that the best detection technology is a combination of your keen eyes and cerebral processing along with clinical experience gained over time!

2.6 Tooth wear: clinical detection

2.6.1 Targeted verbal history

In patients with tooth-wear lesions, it is vital that not only are these detected and a putative cause attributed (i.e. erosive, attritive, or abrasive lesions from their clinical presentation; see later), but also that the aetiology of the erosion/attrition/abrasion is appreciated by both the patient and the oral healthcare team. In this way, the overall clinical problem can be managed successfully. Coupled to the general information obtained from the initial history as discussed previously, more specific questions may be targeted to assess the aetiology of the specific type of tooth wear, often after the initial clinical examination:

- Relating to erosion:
  - past/present diet (using a diet analysis sheet; see Figure 2.19); questions regarding specific acidic food/drinks using an *aide-mémoire* (see Figure 2.20)
  - digestive disorders causing regurgitation erosion/pregnancy sickness

- past/present slimming habits, eating disorders, periods of weight loss
- past/present alcohol intake
- past/present medications (e.g. vitamin C, iron preparations)
- past/present occupation—possibility of industrial erosion, rare nowadays.

- Relating to attrition:
  - clenching/grinding habits—day- or night-time
  - levels of stress/anxiety in personal/professional life
  - evidence of masseteric hypertrophy.

- Relating to abrasion:
  - past/present oral hygiene techniques (tooth brushing, flossing, abrasive pastes)
  - habits that cause dental abrasion—pipe smoking, pen chewing, fingernail biting, etc. (see Figure 2.21).

Table 2.6 Examples of modern technologies available to help detect and characterize carious lesions. The four columns indicate the basic physical principle on which each technology relies. The second row gives the technologies useful in the research laboratory

	OPTICAL/ LIGHT SCATTERING	MINERAL DENSITY	FLUORESCENCE	TISSUE POROSITY
In vivo	Modified ICDAS classification Fibreoptic transillumination UV illumination Quantitative laser fluorescence (QLF) DiagnoDent	Radiography (digital) Radio VisioGraphy Computer tomography (CT) scans (cone beam)	Quantitative laser fluorescence Dye-enhanced laser fluorescence UV illumination DiagnoDent	Electrical conductance measurement (ECM) AC Impedance Dye-enhanced laser fluorescence Dye penetration (iodide) Ultrasound
In vitro	Polarized, transmitted light microscopy (PTLM) Spectroscopy (IR, microRaman) Reflected light confocal microscopy	SEM Quantitative backscattered SEM Microradiography Microfocal CT X-ray microtomography X-ray microanalysis	Confocal laserscanning fluorescence microscopy	Polarized transmission Light microscopy Acoustic microscopy

Name... Number.. Sex   M   F

Address .... Tel no ....

.... Occupation..

.... Work place...

Interests, hobbies, sport activities ....

Medication ....

Illness present .... Illness past ....

Has the illness been treated............................ By a doctor .... In hospital ....

GASTRIC SYMPTOMS	PAST SYMPTOMS			NO	PRESENT SYMPTOMS		
	Frequency per week	Frequency per day	Duration		Frequency per week	Frequency per day	Duration
Belching							
Heartburn							
Acid taste in the mouth							
Vomiting							
Regurgitation ? chew cud							
Stomach ache							
Gastric pain on awakening							
How does the patient treat gastric pain?							

DIET	PAST CONSUMPTION			NO	PRESENT CONSUMPTION		
	Frequency per week	Frequency per day	Duration		Frequency per week	Frequency per day	Duration
Citrus fruits							
Citrus fruit juice							
Other juices							
Special juices							
Sport drinks							
Fruit berries							
Soft drinks, acidic beverages							
Yoghurt							
Vitamin-C drinks, chewable tablets							
Acid sweets							
Special diet							
Vinegar							
Herb tea							
Pickles							
Other acidic food, etc.							
Alcohol							

Figure 2.20 An example of an *aide-mémoire* for use when taking a targeted history for dental erosion.

2.6.2 Clinical presentation of tooth wear

The basic causes of pathological tooth wear (erosion, attrition, abrasion, and abfraction) have been discussed in Chapter 1. The clinical examination outlined in Section 2.4 will permit visual detection of some characteristic features (site/shape of facets/presence of facets on opposing teeth) of the different presentations of tooth wear. However, these are often combined as the cause, and therefore the clinical manifestations, of tooth-wear lesions are multifactorial (see Figure 2.22)

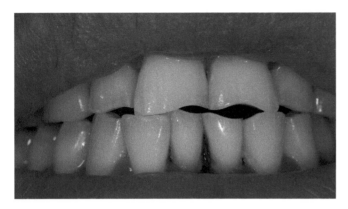

Figure 2.21 An intriguing case of anterior, incisal, undulating abrasion lesions.

Q2.9: What is the cause of the case shown in Figure 2.21?

- *Erosion*: depending on the cause, affects the labial (dietary acids) and palatal smooth surfaces/mandibular buccal/occlusal surfaces (gastric regurgitation acids). Enamel loses its histological surface characterization and becomes smooth and featureless (see Figures 2.23 and 2.24), and eventually grossly dissolves to expose dentine. Can cause smooth-cupped lesions on posterior occlusal surfaces (see Figure 2.24 b).

- *Attrition*: often produces sharp, well-defined, interdigitating tooth-wear lesions on the incisal edges of anterior teeth that meet in occlusion (see Figure 2.23). Can also affect the occlusal surfaces of the molars, but to a lesser extent.

- *Abrasion*: lesions caused by repetitive foreign body contact (e.g. tooth brushing) (classical v-shaped notching on the buccal cervical aspect of mainly anterior teeth).

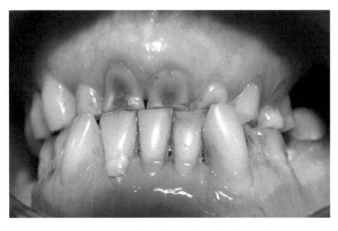

Figure 2.22 A clinical case of tooth wear showing the multifactorial aetiology, including incisal attrition, labial erosion, and buccal cervical abrasion in a middle-aged patient.

Q2.10: What would be the obvious cause of the buccal cervical abrasion shown in Figure 2.22?

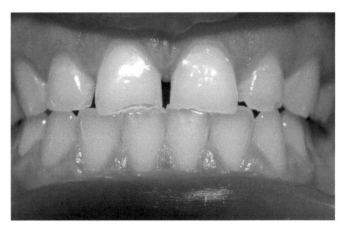

Figure 2.23 A clinical anterior view of a patient with labial–cervical erosion. Note the reflective, smooth, featureless labial enamel surfaces of UR2 and UL2. There are early signs of incisal attrition and the resulting blue-grey translucency.

Q2.11: What might be the presenting complaint of the patient shown in Figure 2.23?

2.6.3 Summary of the clinical manifestations of tooth wear

- The clinical features of faceting/loss of mineralized tissues highlighted in the previous section, cuspal wear (see Figure 2.24b).

- Dental sensitivity/pain caused by active tooth wear as dentine tubules are freshly exposed and pain is elicited on hot and cold stimulation (physiological principles of Brannström's hydrodynamic theory). This is surprisingly uncommon, as tertiary/reparative dentine deposition will often prevent pulp symptoms from occurring.

- Weakened and chipped incisal edges causing trauma to and/or pain from the anterior tip of the tongue (due to roughness), and poor aesthetics (see Figures 2.22 and 2.23).

- Blue-grey appearance of the thinned enamel incisal edges, and possible darkening of teeth due to the change in the optical qualities of the remaining mineralized tissues, again affecting overall aesthetics (see Figure 2.23).

- Loss of tooth structure/fractured teeth or restorations possibly leading to difficulties in chewing due to changes in the occlusion (loss of occlusal contacts, changes in vertical dimension of the bite) and aesthetics (see Figure 2.22).

- Increased risk of marginal fracture/defects of existing restorations as the surrounding hard tissues wear away more rapidly, leaving restorations standing proud.

- Pulpitis, exposure, or even loss of vitality attributable to the extent of tissue loss.

Some of these features may need operative management to provide immediate relief of acute symptoms, or to restore overall dental form and function. However, unless the aetiological factor(s) responsible for tooth wear are discovered, it will never be cured for that particular

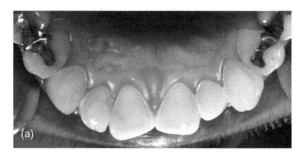 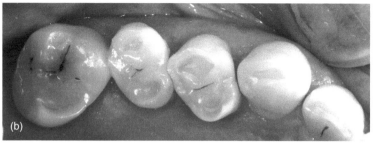

Figure 2.24 (a) A mirrored clinical palatal view of an anterior dentition with erosion caused by excessive consumption of dietary acids. Note the smooth surfaces and peripheral rims of enamel on UL3 to UR3, as well as the amalgam restorations in the premolars standing proud of the tooth surfaces. There was no evidence of gastro-oesophageal reflux from the history. **(b)** A clinical image of the maxillary right quadrant of a patient, showing the cupping lesions associated with dental erosion (with an attritive component as well). ((b) Courtesy of L. Mackenzie.)

patient, and the problems will return (see later). Tooth wear also needs careful reviewing over a prolonged period in order to allow assessment of its relative progress (see Chapter 9). As with caries and periodontal disease, several screening indices exist to enable practitioners to ascertain the level and state of progress of the tooth wear, and the prognosis of any treatment provided, and to undertake medium- to long-term monitoring with careful documentation. One such simple screening tool, the Basic Erosive Wear Examination (BEWE), can be used to stage tooth wear in a similar way to that in which the Basic Periodontal Examination

(BPE) assesses periodontal disease (see Tables 2.7, 2.8, and 2.9, or scan QR code image 2.3).

www.ncbi.
nlm.nih.gov/
pmc/articles/
PMC2238785

QR code image 2.3 Scan this code with your mobile device to view the Basic Erosive Wear Examination tool.

Table 2.7 Clinical sequence to be followed when using the BEWE

1	Diagnose the presence of tooth wear; eliminate teeth with trauma and developmental defects from the score
2	Examine all teeth and all surfaces of teeth in the mouth for tooth wear
3	Identify in each quadrant the most severely affected tooth with wear
4	Calculate the BEWE score

Reprinted by permission from Macmillan Publishers Ltd: *British Dental Journal*, D Bartlett, 'A proposed system for screening tooth wear', 208, 5. c 2010.

Table 2.8 Criteria for grading erosive wear

Score	Features
0	No erosive wear
1	Initial loss of surface texture
2	Distinct defect, hard tissue loss < 50% of the surface area
3	Hard tissue loss ≥ 50% of the surface area

Reprinted by permission from Macmillan Publishers Ltd: *British Dental Journal*, D Bartlett, 'A proposed system for screening tooth wear', 208, 5. © 2010.

Table 2.9 Complexity levels as a guide to clinical management

Complexity level	Cumulative score of all sextants	Management
0	≤ 2	Routine maintenance and observation Repeat at 3-year intervals
1	3–8	Oral hygiene and dietary assessment and advice, routine maintenance and observation Repeat at 2-year intervals

(*continued*)

Table 2.9 (*continued*)

2	9–13	Oral hygiene and dietary assessment and advice, identification of the main aetiological factor(s) responsible for tissue loss, and development of strategies to eliminate respective impacts Consider fluoridation measures or other strategies to increase the resistance of tooth surfaces Ideally, avoid the placement of restorations and monitor erosive wear with study casts, photographs, or silicone impressions Repeat at 6- to 12-month intervals
3	≥ 14	Oral hygiene and dietary assessment and advice, identification of the main aetiological factor(s) responsible for tissue loss, and development of strategies to eliminate respective impacts Consider fluoridation measures or other strategies to increase resistance of tooth surfaces Ideally, avoid restorations and monitor tooth wear with study casts, photographs, or silicone impressions Especially in cases of severe progression, consider special care that may involve restorations Repeat at 6- to 12-month intervals

2.7 Dental trauma: clinical detection

For patients presenting to general dental practice having sustained facial/oral/dental trauma, it is imperative that before any clinical examination is performed, a thorough history is taken of the incident leading to and causing the trauma. Any suspicions of a head injury including facial fractures (from the history, patient behaviour, or general physical examination) should be dealt with by immediate referral to a hospital accident and emergency unit for medical investigation.

Other dentally relevant points to consider are the following:

- *Patient's age*: stage of tooth/root and soft tissue development, and patient compliance issues.
- *Direction of impact/blow/injury*: relevant to the possible direction of displacement of tissues/restorations.
- *Extra-oral soft tissue injuries*: examine cheeks and lip lacerations before investigating intra-orally. Make clear records with diagrams/photographs (after obtaining appropriate consent).

- *Teeth*: can the patient occlude their teeth? Have any teeth been avulsed from their sockets, and if so, for how long and has the patient managed to retrieve the tooth? Tooth displacement (including intrusion), mobility (of the individual tooth or dentoalveolar complex), bleeding from intra-oral soft tissue wounds. Type of dental fracture sustained (see Figure 2.25).

Note that if the interval between the injury and presentation is short, pulp vitality testing and percussion tests will have no diagnostic value, as the teeth are more than likely to have been concussed and the periodontal ligament bruised. Patient compliance during these investigations (including intra-oral radiography) may also be limited! Depending on the severity and symptoms of the injury, it might be worth cleaning up the soft tissue wounds, removing blood clots, performing debridement under local anaesthesia where necessary, and prescribing relevant and necessary antibiotics and pain relief medication at the first visit, and then inviting the patient to return after 2 to 3 days in order to investigate the dental injuries further and initiate a suitably individualized care plan (see later).

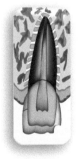 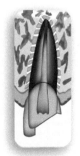 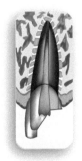 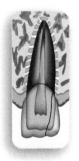 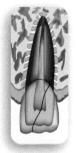 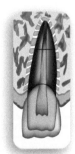

| Enamel infraction
Enamel fracture | Enamel + dentine
fracture | Enamel + dentine
+ pulp fracture
(complicated fracture) | Uncomplicated
crown-root fracture
(enamel + dentine
+ cementum) | Complicated
crown-root
fracture (e +
d + c + pulp) | Root fracture |

Figure 2.25 Classification of traumatic dental tooth fractures. (Reproduced from J D Andreasen et al. *Textbook and Colour Atlas of Traumatic Injuries to Teeth*, Fourth Edition. © 2007, with permission from John Wiley & Sons Ltd.)

2.8 Developmental defects

As teeth develop and form they are at risk of developing defects that manifest clinically after tooth eruption, often affecting tooth size/shape/number or the quality/quantity of the mineralized tissues themselves. These affected teeth can pose an aesthetic problem, and may also be more prone to the ravages of tooth wear and/or carious attack. These defects have to be detected and diagnosed from the intra-oral dental examination and careful history taking, especially of childhood or maternal illnesses or trauma to the deciduous dentition. Although developmental defects are relatively rare, the aetiology and clinical appearance of some of the more commonly occurring ones have been described in Table 2.10.

Table 2.10 Developmental defects categorized as acquired and hereditary, with descriptions of their basic aetiology and clinical appearance

Developmental defect		Aetiology	Clinical appearance
Acquired	Enamel hypoplasia (see Figure 2.26)	Ameloblast damage (systemic childhood infectious diseases, trauma/infection to deciduous predecessor)	
		Hypoplastic: ↓ matrix, normal maturation	Pitted, thin enamel of normal hardness
		Hypomineralized: normal matrix, ↓ mineralization	Opaque, chalky-white, ?softened enamel
		Systemic cause	Defined areas, bands on all teeth developing at time of illness
	Molar–incisor hypomineralization (see Figure 2.27)	Systemic illness (high fever, respiratory illness) from 0 to 2 years affecting occlusal surfaces of the first molars and possibly maxillary incisors	
		Hypomineralized	White-yellow or yellow-brown opacities, easily chipped, ↑ sensitivity (exposed dentine, plaque stagnation)
	Intrinsic dental fluorosis (see Figure 2.28)	Excessive fluoride ion intake (water, toothpaste, tablets) poisons ameloblast function during enamel formation/maturation	Chalky-white flecks, confluent blotches, brown discoloration, pitted enamel
	Intrinsic tetracycline stain (see Figure 2.29)	Broad-spectrum antibiotic with affinity for mineralized tissues. If taken by mother during pregnancy, deciduous teeth are affected; if taken at age < 12 years, permanent teeth are affected. Rare nowadays	Dark grey horizontal bands affecting all teeth
Hereditary (genetic, familial history)	Hypodontia (oligodontia)	Some teeth do not develop; associated with microdontia. Third molars, second premolars, and upper lateral incisors most affected	Abnormal crown shape/size
	Amelogenesis imperfecta (see Figure 2.30)	Abnormalities in enamel formation (complex classification)	
		Hypoplastic: defect of matrix formation	Thin enamel, yellowish teeth (dentine showing through). Or granular, pitted, stained thin enamel
		Hypomineralized and hypomature: defective matrix mineralization and maturation	Soft, friable, stained, or chalky-white enamel, frequently lost due to weakness at the enamel–dentine junction (EDJ)
	Dentinogenesis imperfecta	Odontoblast defect affecting dentine matrix formation and mineralization. Rare	Enamel lost rapidly due to defective EDJ. Brown, opalescent dentine colour, prone to fracture/wear. Short roots, bulbous crowns, pulps obliterated

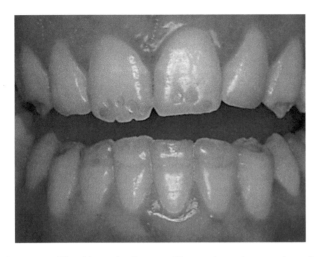

Figure 2.26 Pitted hypoplastic enamel in a patient who experienced a severe childhood illness. Note the pattern of teeth affected—maxillary central incisors and tips of maxillary canines and all mandibular incisors approximately a third of the length from the incisal edges and tips of the mandibular canines too.

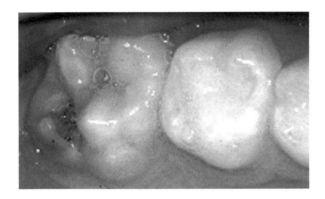

Figure 2.27 Example of molar hypomineralization with yellow-brown opacities on the occlusal surface of UR6. The disto-palatal fissure shows marked enamel breakdown and demarcated border opacities. (Courtesy of K. Weerheijm.)

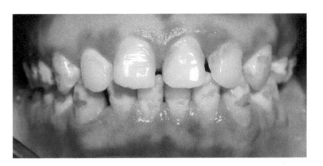

Figure 2.28 Severe dental fluorosis with characteristic generalized enamel pitting and brown discoloration. This patient resided in a Sudanese village with natural fluoride levels in the drinking water exceeding 4000 ppm F. The maxillary central incisors have been polished by a dentist using a fine grit bur, so removing the superficial weakened fluorotic enamel.

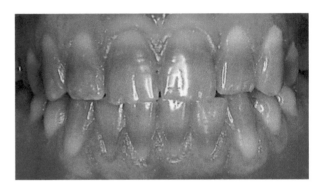

Figure 2.29 Severe intrinsic tetracycline staining with classic horizontal banding of the stain on the labial surfaces.

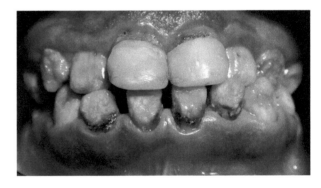

Figure 2.30 Severe hypoplastic amelogenesis imperfecta with hard, thin, and pitted enamel remaining on the teeth. The patient presented with two poor-quality acrylic crowns on the upper central incisors, and buccal cervical caries on the lower incisors.

2.9 Suggested further reading and PubMed keywords

Andreasen JO, Andreasen FM, Andersson L. (eds) (2007) *Textbook and Colour Atlas of Traumatic Injuries to Teeth*, 4th edn. Oxford: Blackwell Munksgaard.
<http://eu.wiley.com/WileyCDA/WileyTitle/pro-ductCd-1405129549.html>

www.ncbi.nlm.nih.gov/pubmed/advanced

QR code image 2.4 Try searching the following keywords on PubMed for relevant further reading. You can access PubMed by scanning the QR code image or at the address

Keywords

ICDAS; cariogram; CAMBRA; Previser

2.10 Answers to self-test questions

Q2.1: Can you spot an error in the charting in Figure 2.2?

A: In the LL5, there is no MO charted in 'existing restorations', but one has been included in 'treatment to be done.' Well spotted!

Q2.2: What hand instrument should be used instead and for what purpose?

A: A blunt, round-headed dental explorer/periodontal probe.

Q2.3: What treatment may be required for the tooth shown in Figure 2.8?

A: Initial improvement in oral hygiene to remove the plaque effectively from the occlusal surface. If the patient is not compliant, a disto-occlusal restoration may be required.

Q2.4: Can you find more lesions in Figure 2.14 (a) and (b) and classify them radiographically? Can you comment on the radiographic changes of the pulp chambers in those teeth?

A: Mesial UR6, distal UR5: D1—note how even in these relatively distant lesions, tertiary dentine has partly occluded the pulp chambers in these teeth.

Q2.5: What is the cause of the radiolucencies in Figure 2.14 (c)? (Clue—look carefully at (d) for the answer!)

A: The well-defined occlusal radiolucency is caused by superimposition of the radiolucent resin composite restoration that is evident buccally. The proximal radiolucencies are cervical burnout, due to the narrowing of the tooth at this morphological junction between crown and root.

Q2.6:

i. Can you guess which materials have been used to restore the cavity in the maxillary molar in Figure 2.14 (e)?

ii. What other information would you need before deciding to operatively intervene or not, to manage the diffuse radiolucency subjacent to the restoration?

iii. What might be the cause of the radio-opacity in the mandibular molar?

A:

i. The more radio-opaque overlying material is probably a resin composite. The underlying less radio-opaque material is possibly a GIC or Biodentine (see Chapter 7).

ii. The clinical findings with regard to the integrity of the proximal margin, signs/symptoms from the patient/pulp, pulp tests, presence of caries elsewhere in the mouth, review of previous notes/radiographs.

iii. The presence of a resin composite restoration (preventive resin restoration; see Chapter 8).

Q2.7: How could you manage the case shown in Figure 2.18?

A: Improve oral hygiene and minimally restore the cavity to enable easier biofilm removal.

Q2.8: What stands out as the main problem regarding the sugar intake of the patient in Figure 2.19?

A: The number of episodes per day and their frequency throughout each 24-hour period. This would ensure that the patient's teeth were bathed in plaque with a pH below 5.5 for significant periods, leading to demineralization of the enamel.

Q2.9: What is the cause of the case shown in Figure 2.21?

A: The patient plays with a large, metal tongue stud across the anterior teeth, causing a significant amount of tooth-wear damage.

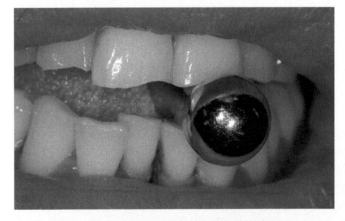

Q2.10: What would be the obvious cause of the buccal cervical abrasion shown in Figure 2.22?

A: Excessive or prolonged action of horizontal tooth brushing.

Q2.11: What might be the presenting complaint of the patient shown in Figure 2.23?

A: The appearance of the incisal edges, chipping of the front teeth, sharpness to the tongue, grey discoloration.

3

Diagnosis, prognosis, and care planning: 'information processing'

Chapter contents

3.1 Introduction

Once a general and targeted history, examination, and investigations have been carried out ('information gathering'), it is time for the dentist and their oral healthcare team to assimilate all of the relevant information in order to formulate a diagnosis, prognosis, and care plan for the individual patient ('information processing'). Although the detection and diagnostic phases are each discussed separately in this book, an experienced clinician will often accomplish both phases simultaneously. It is vital to remember that *diagnosis precedes treatment* in all cases.

3.1.1 Definitions

Diagnosis

Diagnosis is the art or act of inferring, from its signs and symptoms or manifestations, the nature or cause of an illness or condition. This stage is critical in order to allow the dental team and the patient to appreciate the nature, cause, and severity of the illness or condition.

Prognosis

The prognosis is the forecast of the course of a disease or the patient's response to treatment of the disease. This stage helps the dentist and the patient to understand how easy or difficult the treatment will be to carry out, and it allows assessment of the patient's motivation to cure the problem. In dentistry, the oral healthcare team can only start the patient off on the road to recovery by restoring form and function to their dentition as well as helping the patient to prevent or control the disease process, so preventing its return. It is then up to the patient whether they follow this advice and maintain their oral health in the future.

Patient-centred care plan

This plan is the formal itemized management strategy, developed by the dentist and their oral healthcare team, for the individual patient to treat the manifestations of a disease and to control it or prevent it from recurring. It can be divided into *phases* of therapy (e.g. prevention or control, stabilization or definitive treatment, and review, reassessment, or recall), and it should be adapted and modified during its execution for maximum benefit to the patient. It should take into account unforeseen developments in the course of the disease or the patient's response to care. It should be written down and made clear to all parties for discussion, so that informed consent can be gained prior to implementation.

3.2 Diagnosing dental pain, or 'toothache'

'Common diseases occur commonly.' A list of common diagnoses of dental pain follows, and the various features of each are summarized in Table 3.1.

- Acute pulpitis.
- Acute periapical periodontitis.
- Acute periapical abscess.
- Acute periodontal (lateral) abscess.
- Chronic pulpitis.
- Chronic periapical periodontitis (apical granuloma).
- Exposed sensitive dentine.
- Interproximal food packing.
- Cracked cusps/tooth syndrome.

Other conditions which are beyond the remit of this book and that may also manifest as dento-facial pain include maxillary sinusitis, trigeminal neuralgia, facial arthromyalgia, and pericoronitis. It must be understood that pain symptoms rarely fall neatly into the diagnoses listed previously (see also Table 3.1), and that a degree of clinical experience will be required to interpret the relevant signs and symptoms and thus permit a diagnosis to be made. It is important to recognize that the signs and symptoms from an inflamed pulp do not necessarily correlate fully with the histological changes that are occurring within that pulp. Therefore all interpretation of the signs and symptoms must be undertaken with caution.

3.2.1 Acute pulpitis

- Acute, severe, poorly localized pain.
- Does not cross the facial midline, and might be difficult for the patient to identify from which jaw it is originating. They may present holding their face on the relevant side, rather than identifying a particular tooth.
- There are two clinical presentations (not necessarily relating to pulp histology), *reversible* and *irreversible*. Table 3.2 highlights their similarities and differences.
- Clinically, offending teeth may present with carious lesions or large restorations which may be defective, but the dentist must always check the status of the dentition in both quadrants on the relevant side.

3.2.2 Acute periapical periodontitis

- Pain localizable to the offending tooth—the patient will be able to point to it and will complain of pain when biting on it (due to stimulation of pain- and pressure-sensitive fibres in the periodontal ligament).
- Tooth tender to palpation and percussion. This should only entail a gentle pushing action on suspect teeth into their sockets or laterally. It does not mean tapping the crown of the tooth with a mirror handle

Table 3.1 Classic signs and symptoms for differential diagnoses for dental pain (unfortunately, not all symptoms fall within these clear categories, and experience is required when interpreting them)

	Acute pulpitis	Acute apical periodontitis	Acute apical abscess	Acute periodontal abscess	Exposed sensitive dentine	Food packing	Cracked cusp	Chronic pulpitis	Chronic apical periodontitis (apical granuloma)
History	Recent pain with hot and cold stimuli. May be very severe. Poorly localized	Tender to bite. Well localized	Pain and swelling Very well localized	Localized swelling. Some pain	Generalized pain in response to hot, cold, and sweet stimuli	Pain after eating fibrous food, e.g. meat	Vague intermittent pain usually on biting. May be poorly localized	Vague, unprovoked intermittent but increasing pain. Poorly localized	May have had pain in the past. Now not sensitive to hot and cold
Clinical examination	Possibly caries or recent large restoration	Possibly caries	May be extra-oral or intra-oral swelling over apex of tooth	intra-oral swelling nearer to gingival margin. Tooth may be mobile	Gingival recession. Exposed dentine at the gingival margin. Sensitive to probe or cold air	Open contact points. Gingival inflammation. Food usually present	Often nothing, but crack may be seen. May be painful with occlusal contact only	May have large restoration or caries	May have large restoration or caries
Vitality test	Hypersensitive	May still be vital, but usually non-vital	Non-vital	Often vital	Vital	May be vital or non-vital	May be hypersensitive	Often normal but may be hypersensitive	Non-vital
Percussion	Not tender	Tender	Tender to touch. Too tender to percuss	Slight tenderness, more to lateral than axial pressure	Not tender	Not tender to percussion. May be sore with lateral percussion	Usually not tender but may be	Not tender	Slightly. May give dull sound on percussion
Other clinical tests			Raised temperature. Looks ill	Deep pockets. Pus may be released on probing pocket		Floss passes the contact easily	Sometimes tender to lateral pressure on an individual cusp		
Radiographic findings	Probably caries close to pulp. No periapical change	Usually no periapical change in early stage	Usually no periapical change except slight thickening of apical periodontal membrane	Alveolar bone loss. Usually no periapical change	May be some alveolar bone loss	None	None	None	Periapical radiolucency
Findings on further investigations	Carious exposure of pulp	Necrotic pulp	Pus may be drained via abscess cavity to root canal without local anaesthetic, giving immediate relief of pain and confirming the diagnosis				Crack sometimes visible at base of cavity when old restoration is removed. If left, cuspal fracture will eventually occur	Symptoms may settle if restoration is removed and tooth is dressed with calcium hydroxide, but pulp often dies eventually	Necrotic pulp

Table 3.2 Characteristics of acute pulpitis

Reversible pulpitis	Irreversible pulpitis
• Characteristic short, sharp pain	• Characteristic dull, throbbing pain (although the patient may experience bouts of sharp pain)
• *Stimulated* by hot, cold, or sweet stimuli	• Onset is usually unprovoked/ *exacerbated* by hot, cold, or sweet stimuli
• *A few seconds*; *disappears* when stimulus is removed	• *Several minutes to several hours*; *persists* when stimulus is removed
• Pulp sensibility tests may elicit an exaggerated response	• Pulp sensibility tests may elicit an exaggerated or negative response
• Tooth is not tender to percussion (TTP)	• Tooth is not TTP (except in late-stage presentation)

(warn the patient that this examination may be uncomfortable, and obtain their permission before you undertake it).

• Tenderness felt over the root apex through mucosae in the buccal sulcus.

• Pulp may initially retain vitality, but will eventually become necrotic.

• Periapical radiograph *may* show loss of lamina dura around the root apex region during late-stage presentation.

3.2.3 Acute periapical abscess

• Patient may present with a large facial and/or intra-oral swelling associated with the affected relevant quadrant, or a more localized swelling in the alveolar mucosa over the affected root.

• May present before swelling occurs, or after it has burst and subsided, with evidence of a sinus tract.

• Patient may present with fever.

• Tooth will be painful to bite on; negative results with vitality tests (if permitted).

• Periapical radiograph will usually show loss of lamina dura and widening of the periodontal ligament space around the root apex.

3.2.4 Acute periodontal (lateral) abscess

• Forms at the base of a deep periodontal pocket.

• Well-localized pain associated with a vital pulp.

• If this is combined with pulpal necrosis (of differing aetiology), a 'perio-endo' lesion can be diagnosed, often with a poor prognosis, leading to extraction of the tooth.

3.2.5 Chronic pulpitis

• Mild, poorly localized, periodic, grumbling pain (on and off) over several weeks or months.

• Initially vital pulp and tooth not tender to percussion, but if condition progresses, symptoms of periapical periodontitis may eventually supervene.

• Initial treatment will involve monitoring to assess whether the pulp has recovered after treating the cause (e.g. caries, cracked tooth).

• More severe cases will require removal of any restoration, placement of a sedative dressing over the pulp, and then a provisional restoration.

3.2.6 Chronic periapical periodontitis

• Can be symptomless or may elicit mild pain on biting.

• Positive response to vigorous percussion, or even presentation with a sinus tract (see Figure 3.1).

• Periapical radiograph shows well-demarcated radiolucency around the root apex (see Figure 3.2).

• Often described as an apical granuloma.

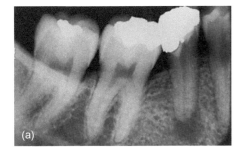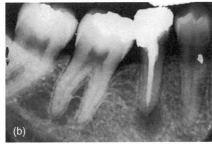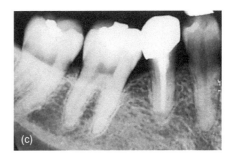

Figure 3.1 (a) Periapical radiograph showing a well-demarcated radiolucency at the apex of LR5 (with accompanying loss of lamina dura and relative widening of the periodontal ligament space when compared with the adjacent healthy LR7). The large restoration has contributed to pulp necrosis in this tooth, and it is likely that a periapical granuloma has formed, but this should strictly be diagnosed from histological analysis of a biopsy sample. **(b)** Periapical radiograph of the same tooth after the gutta-percha root filling was placed. **(c)** Radiograph taken 3 years later, showing healing around the root apex of the LR5, bony infill, and re-formed lamina dura. (Courtesy of the late Professor Pitt Ford.)

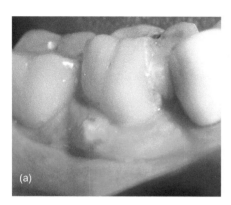
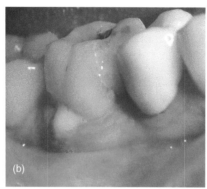
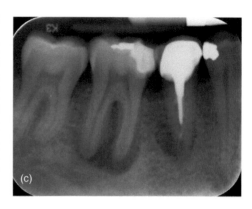

Figure 3.2 Chronically infected apical granuloma **(a)** with pus pointing through a sinus on the mucosa adjacent to the non-vital LR6 **(b)**. **(c)** Periapical radiograph shows a large radiolucency associated with the apices and furcation of the LR6, as well as a separate periapical radiolucency on the heavily restored (but inadequately root-treated) LR5.

- The apical granuloma is a chronic inflammatory response (highly vascularized granulation tissue) to toxins leaching from the necrotic pulp and causing increased osteoclastic action in the subjacent bone, leading to bone resorption. As the toxins become diluted, the extent of the resorption is naturally limited. If the necrotic pulp, and therefore the source of toxins, is removed, bony repair can result (see Figure 3.2).

- If infection occurs, the chronic apical granuloma can flare up into an acute apical abscess with sinus tract (see Figure 3.1).

- Chronic apical granulomas may become cystic and require treatment by surgical intervention (see Figure 3.3).

3.2.7 Exposed sensitive dentine

- Poorly localized short, sharp sensitivity to hot, cold, or sweet stimuli, caused by exposed root dentine surfaces (gingival recession, root

caries). The pain response can be elicited by air-drying the exposed surface using a dental 3-1 air/water syringe.

- Positive pulp test (perhaps slightly hyper-responsive if tested during an acute episode), and teeth not tender to percussion.

- To reduce the sensitivity, the exposed tubules may be blocked using a dentine bonding agent or a thin layer of resin composite. Use of potassium nitrate/chloride compounds may help to reduce tubule conduction and pain transmission.

3.2.8 Interproximal food packing

- Open contact point (drifted teeth, poor contouring of adjacent proximal restorations) enables food debris to get caught between teeth and traumatize the interdental gingival papillae, leading to localized tenderness, bleeding, and inflammation.

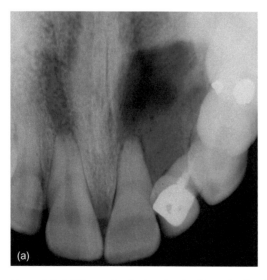
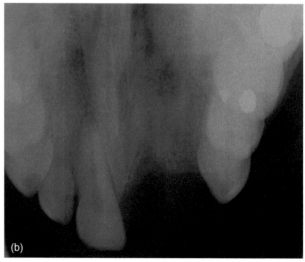

Figure 3.3 (a) Upper standard occlusal radiographs showing large palatal cystic change in an apical granuloma associated with UL12. **(b)** The same radiograph taken 3 years later after UL12 had been extracted and the cyst surgically managed. Note the near complete bony infill of the initially large defect. Implants were placed successfully into the new bone to restore UL12.

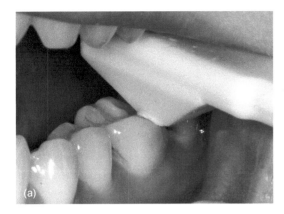
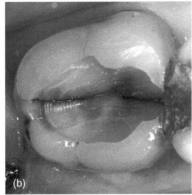
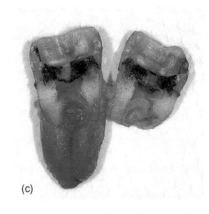

Figure 3.4 (a) A Tooth Slooth® (sleuth) detects whether there is a cracked cusp on the disto-buccal aspect of the left mandibular first molar. The patient bites on the plastic tip, which directs the occlusal force on to the disto-buccal cusp in this case. Pain may be elicited on pressure or on release as the cracked cusp flexes under occlusal strain. **(b)** A mandibular molar with symptoms of a cracked tooth. The large existing amalgam restoration was removed, revealing a clear fracture line mesio-distally (more easily detected using magnification; see Chapter 5, Section 5.7). As the portions of the tooth were mobile and the coronal extent of the fracture was considerable, the tooth was deemed unrestorable and it was extracted. **(c)** The subgingival extent of the oblique shear fracture, through the pulp chamber. (Courtesy of L. Mackenzie.)

3.2.9 Cracked cusp/tooth syndrome

- Cracks can involve enamel only (no pain, similar to superficial cracks in a porcelain teacup), or enamel and dentine (which may or may not include the pulp), which can cause poorly localized pain periodically.

- There is sometimes a sharp pain on biting/thermal stimulus. Pulp tests may be inconclusive, as may percussion and palpation tests.

- Transillumination or dyes can be used to detect cracks, but do not relate their presence to the cause of pain.

- Diagnostic testing may involve careful analysis of pain on biting. Using a cotton-wool roll, wood stick (wooden tongue depressor split lengthways), rubber suction tip, or proprietary kits (e.g. Tooth Slooth®), cracked tooth/cusp pain can be elicited on specific cusps, at specific angles of pressure, and assessed both on biting and release. This helps to ascertain where and how deep the crack might be, and thus what treatment is required (see Figure 3.4).

3.3 Caries risk/susceptibility assessment

The aetiology and histopathology of caries, as well as the methods for detecting it, have been discussed in Chapters 1 and 2. Once this information has been gathered through a targeted verbal history and examination, analysis ('information processing') is required to ascertain the risk and likelihood of the individual patient developing further disease and responding to treatment of current disease. This is achieved by relating the risk status of the patient on presentation to the activity state of any lesions present. This is known as a caries risk/susceptibility assessment or analysis. Without this knowledge, caries management at the individual patient level will never be successful in the long term. Risk assessments can also be carried out at a population level in order to help to promote public health prevention strategies for large numbers of people (e.g. water fluoridation programmes).

- It makes economic and practical sense to target preventive treatments in practice at the appropriate risk group.

- Dental care neither begins nor ends with a single course of treatment, but is ongoing. When a course of dental treatment is complete, the dentist, team, and patient decide when it would be wise to check that all is well. This recall interval is based partly on an assessment

of the likelihood and risk of disease progression, and should not be standardized at 6 months or any other period.

- The patient must be made aware of their risk status. This knowledge encourages them to attend appropriately timed recall appointments, to become motivated and involved, taking responsibility for their own preventive care, and, if they pay for their treatment, it may help them to budget for dental bills.

The various patient factors that affect the risk assessment have been highlighted in Table 3.3. The relevance of these factors in a targeted verbal history of risk assessment has been indicated in Table 2.1 (in Chapter 2), and a chart similar to Table 3.4 might be used in the patient notes to document such findings. Formal, 'standardized' risk assessment systems exist which help the oral healthcare team to calculate their patients' risk status (e.g. Cariogram, Caries Management by Risk Assessment (CAMBRA), PreViser™; QR codes images 3.1 and 3.2 will take you to further information on these systems). In some cases, algorithms are used to process the findings from the patient assessment, giving extra weight and relevance to certain factors that are deemed more important to the risk outcome. Although these can be convenient and helpful

QR Code image 3.1 Scan this code with your mobile device to view the Cariogram risk assessment system.

www.mah.
se/fakulteter-
och-omraden/
Odontologiska-
fakulteten/
Avdelning-
och-kansli/
Cariologi/
Cariogram

QR Code image 3.2 Scan this code with your mobile device to view the PreViser™ risk assessment system.

www.
previser.
co.uk

for teaching and research purposes, there is a risk that the analysis will become too standardized and the nuances and variations for each patient will not be fully appreciated or understood, especially at general practice level. It is more important for the dentist and the oral health-care team to tailor the risk assessment for each patient, with the team and the patient appreciating and understanding fully the relevance and significance of all the information gathered for that specific individual. With the increase in litigation against dentists, risk assessments that are interpreted and recorded formally in the clinical notes are becoming essential dento-legal requirements, not forgetting the obvious ethical

Table 3.3 Factors involved in assessing caries risk and categorizing the patient's susceptibility to caries as high or low risk*

Caries risk assessment

	High risk	Low risk
Social history	Socially deprived	Middle class
	High caries in siblings	Low caries in siblings
	Low knowledge of dental disease	Dentally aware
	Irregular attender	Regular attender
	Ready availability of snacks	Work does not allow regular snacks
	Low dental aspirations	High dental aspirations
Medical history	Medically compromised	No medical problem
	Disabled	No physical problem
	Xerostomia	Normal salivary flow
	Long-term cariogenic medicine	No long-term medication
Dietary habits	Frequent sugar intake	Infrequent sugar intake
Fluoride use	Non-fluoride area	Fluoridation area
	No fluoride supplements	Fluoride supplements used
	No fluoride toothpaste	Fluoride toothpaste used
Plaque control	Infrequent, ineffective cleaning	Frequent/effective cleaning
	Poor manual control	Good manual control
Saliva	Low flow rate	Normal flow rate
	Low buffering capacity	High buffering capacity
	High *Streptococcus mutans* and Lactobacillus counts	Low *S. mutans* and lactobacillus counts
Clinical evidence	New lesions	No new lesions
	Premature extractions	Nil extractions for caries
	Anterior caries or restorations	Sound anterior teeth
	Multiple restorations	No or few restorations
	History of repeated restorations	Restorations inserted years ago
	No fissure sealants	Fissure sealed
	Multiband orthodontics	No appliances
	Partial dentures	

*This information can be gathered from a targeted verbal history and examination (see Chapter 2).

Table 3.4 An example of a chart for noting down key findings from the patient's history and examination in order to help to evaluate their caries risk

Status	'Yes' answer: high risk	'No' answer: low risk
Lesions: Two or more new, progressing, and/or restored lesions in the last 2 years? Activity state?		
General factors		
Diet: Frequent snacks between meals? Anorexia or bulimia? Prolonged nursing/bottle feeding?		
Fluoride: Deficient fluoride exposure (toothpaste/rinse daily, community water fluoridation)?		
Health: Sjögren's syndrome, chemotherapy, radiation to head and neck?		
Medications: Hypo-salivatory medication, polypharmacy?		
Social: Socio-economic status? Parents/siblings with active caries? Symptom-driven attendance?		
Age: Adolescent? Elderly?		
Oral factors		
Oral hygiene: Quality? What aids are used?		
Saliva: Stimulated saliva flow < 0.7 mL/min? pH/buffering capacity?		
Plaque: Readily visible heavy plaque—plaque scores?		
Bacterial balance: Levels of *Streptococcus mutans*		

First published in the *Journal of Minimum Intervention Dentistry* 2009; 2: 103–24. Reproduced here with permission.

dimension to this best practice. The caries risk assessment will change over time, and should therefore be undertaken when the pattern of disease presentation changes in the same patient—the overall patient management of caries is as dynamic as the disease process itself.

With regard to the number of lesions detected during the clinical oral examination, a patient at high risk for caries is one who presents with or has a history of two or more new, progressing, and/or restored carious lesions in the previous 2 years. The patient's caries risk is classified generally into three categories—high, medium, or low (or red, amber, or green (RAG) traffic lights). Although this is useful for epidemiological and research purposes, it can add an unnecessary layer of complexity, or even ambiguity, for the oral healthcare team when assessing patients in general dental practice. A simpler division into low or high risk/susceptibility is usually more than sufficient to paint the individual risk picture for the patient, and aids the formulation of their individualized care plan accordingly. It is of course recognized that there are patient subgroups within the general population who are susceptible to certain factors (e.g. radiotherapy, autoimmune conditions) that elevate their risk to an extreme level (also classified as high risk with unmodifiable factors), and these individuals may require periodic referral for advice about care planning, and indeed may sometimes need care in a specialist environment (see Chapter 4, Section 4.2.1).

3.4 Diagnosing tooth wear

The detection and diagnosis of tooth wear from its causative factors have been discussed in detail in Chapter 2. A targeted verbal history coupled with rigorous examination of the teeth is essential for reaching a diagnosis of this common multifactorial problem. Differentiating between acceptable age-related and pathological levels of wear can be difficult, as this depends on the patient's age, dental history, and the rate of progress of the tooth wear, which can be difficult to assess clinically unless the patient is reviewed annually in the first instance. However, wear facets with staining or dental plaque present may be indicative of a very slow or arrested rate of progress, whereas significant dental sensitivity from such lesions may indicate a more rapid rate of wear, as there would not have been enough time for the up-regulated odontoblasts to lay down translucent or tertiary dentine (see Chapter 1, Section 1.2.8).

3.5 Diagnosing dental trauma and developmental defects

Again, as with tooth wear, the degree of separation between detection and diagnosis of trauma and developmental defects is negligible, as the two processes are linked intimately with the verbal history and the oral/dental examination. These have been discussed in detail in Chapter 2.

3.6 Prognostic indicators

The dentist should give the patient a verbal and written prognosis of their responsibilities and the potential outcomes of preventive care, the individual tooth or teeth requiring interventional treatment, and/or a prognosis for the management of the overall condition. At the tooth level, factors that affect the prognosis include:

- *Restorability*—that is, the severity of damage incurred to the coronal hard tissues (extent of the carious lesion, and amount of tooth structure lost due to trauma, tooth wear, or developmental defect). Can operative treatment be used to repair and reinstate the tooth structure successfully in the mid to long term?
- The status of the pulp.
- The status of the periodontium (alveolar bone levels, periodontal ligament).

With regard to the underlying condition, prognostic factors include:

- The ease with which the aetiological factors can be removed or modified to prevent or slow the progress of the disease and its recurrence. For example, the aetiology of xerostomia caused by radiation therapy cannot be modified, so dental conditions (e.g. caries) will generally have a poor prognosis. However, with the judicious use of oral hygiene procedures to a high standard, complemented with high concentrations of fluoride, the prognosis may be improved.
- The overall level of patient motivation to manage the condition. If the patient is not particularly concerned or does not wish to take responsibility for maintaining their oral health, the long-term outlook for treatment administered by the oral healthcare team will be bleak at best, and only repairs can be considered. This, together with the long-term consequences of further tooth destruction, must be made clear to the patient and documented fully in the clinical notes.

3.7 Formulating an individualized care plan

3.7.1 Why is a care plan necessary?

The need for and importance of making individualized, adaptable holistic plans (both simple and complex), and of recording the decisions in the patient's clinical record, can be summarized as follows:

- It ensures that the lead clinician reviews the care in the light of all available evidence at the start of treatment and at intervals throughout treatment.
- It is a record for later reference, particularly in complicated cases and after a lapse of time during the treatment period. This is available primarily for the benefit of the patient, but on occasion, when a patient makes a complaint, it will have dento-legal importance and may protect the dentist and their team against unjustified complaints. In this context, when the care plan is complex and expensive, it is essential to put the advice in the form of a letter to the patient so that he or she has time to consider it, is able to digest it and its implications, and has an opportunity to question it before accepting or rejecting it. This process of two-way communication between the dentist and their team and the patient is of critical importance. The

vast majority (more than 90%) of all dento-legal litigation pursued in the UK in 2013 was blamed on poor communication or understanding between the two parties, lack of management of patients' expectations, or inadequate record-keeping. In the UK the General Dental Council now suggests that this formalized two-way approach to planning is recommended practice in all cases.

- It avoids the risk of disorderly and ill-advised treatment, which may occur if treatment is administered piecemeal or by different members of the oral healthcare team or different specialists.

Written care plans, however simple, should be drawn up for every patient. They should be tailored specifically to the individual patient's holistic needs, must take all factors into consideration from the detection and diagnostic phases, and must have realistic goals and be achievable for the dentist, the oral healthcare team, and the patient. They must also be planned by the dentist and their team in such a way as to manage patient expectations with regard to the quality and success of any potential outcome of care. They must include all aspects of care, including non-operative preventive care and recall strategy, rather than just being a list of specific surgical procedures performed by the dentist to treat symptoms of the disease. This is why the traditional 'treatment-plan' terminology is dated and inappropriate clinically. All too often such treatment plans became a shopping list of procedures to be carried out, rather than outlining—with reasons—the purpose of the different phases of care and how they interlink with the responsibilities of the oral healthcare team, the dentist, and the patient to secure a successful outcome.

Patients must understand the implications of the treatment and appreciate that the care plan may deviate from the initial path as the care progresses. They must also acknowledge their own pivotal role in its ultimate success, the time frame for its delivery, and its cost (if applicable).

3.7.2 Structure of the care plan

However simple a care plan may be for a particular management episode, it is wise to have a structure to follow. One such scheme is outlined in Table 3.5, and consists of three phases:

- an initial *stabilization phase* (which may take several months to complete, depending on the amount and type of work required)

- a *reassessment phase*—to re-evaluate the response to the initial treatment, and the future needs of the patient (which may have changed since the time of presentation)

- a *rehabilitation phase*—in which definitive restorations can be designed and placed.

Other considerations include the type of restorative material that is to be used (see Chapter 7), and whether operative intervention will be minimally invasive or more extensive (i.e. whether to restore or attempt to arrest a carious lesion in dentine, restore or monitor an erosive tooth-wear lesion, or extract or endodontically treat an infected tooth). These decisions must be made with input from the patient (including their own perceived need, aesthetic considerations, the number of appointments necessary, costs, and the level of dental anxiety, i.e. appreciating and managing the patient's expectations) as this will confer ownership and therefore responsibility to the patient in terms of the success of the final outcome. Second opinions from more experienced specialists (either practice or hospital based) can be very helpful, especially for the more complex cases, as there is rarely a single right or wrong decision to be made in care planning. Choosing the best of several options for the patient is a skill that develops with further clinical experience, and unfortunately this will involve making some errors of judgement along the way! It is interesting to note that these 'errors of judgement' rarely give rise to formal dento-legal action by patients, so long as the patient

Table 3.5 A care plan flowchart that structures patient care into three phases, which can blend into one another depending on the complexity of the plan.

Care plan phase	Comments
Stabilization	Pain relief ↓ Control active disease Prevention Extraction of teeth with hopeless prognosis Temporary/transitional restorations ↓
Reassessment	Reassess the patient's response to the stabilization phase, their subsequent needs, aesthetic expectations, motivation, dental examination, and costs ↓
Rehabilitation	Reorganizing or conforming to existing occlusal scheme (see later); definitive restorations/prostheses ↓ Review, reassess, and recall (maintenance)

has been involved in the journey and the decision making. Good communication and documentation is the key. Always be prepared to *justify* the successful care plan to three parties—the patient, yourself, and a lawyer! It is vital to learn from these situations and adapt your own evidence base accordingly in the future.

Table 4.1 (in Chapter 4) gives an example of a care plan flowchart for patients with dental caries. It is based on five possible management options, dependent on the presence or absence of active lesions coupled with the individual's caries risk assessment (the overall caries matrix). Of course, real life is not always that simple, and patients' conditions do not always fit within such clear-cut categories, but this concept mapping exercise helps the dentist and the patient to understand the options and where the chosen management strategy fits in relation to the alternatives.

3.8 PubMed keywords

<www.ncbi.nlm.nih.gov/pubmed/advanced>

QR code image 3.3 Try searching the following keywords on PubMed for relevant further reading. You can access PubMed by scanning the QR code image or at the address

Keywords

Basic Erosive Wear Examination (BEWE); Smith and Knight Tooth Wear Index.

4

Disease control and lesion prevention

4.1 Introduction

From the previous chapter it can be seen that in all cases of caries and tooth wear, minimum intervention disease control and lesion prevention are key aspects of the management strategy, often commencing in the stabilization phase of the care plan, but continuing throughout the full course of treatment and beyond in order to maintain lifelong oral health.

4.1.1 Disease control

Neither the dentist, as part of the oral healthcare team, nor the patient has the power to *prevent* the caries or tooth-wear process. These ubiquitous processes occur at the ionic, metabolic, and microscopic level at the tooth surface/biofilm interface, and are made pathological by other factors in combination. If these factors are controlled or modified by the patient (with help from the oral healthcare team), then the processes can be regulated. The term *primary prevention* is sometimes used in this context.

4.1.2 Lesion prevention

The term *prevention* has been commonly used, but actually it is only the manifestation of the pathological process (i.e. the lesion in caries or tooth wear) that can be prevented if the disease process is controlled. The term *secondary prevention* has been used in this context to slow down or stop (arrest) incipient, progressing lesions. *Tertiary prevention* is a term sometimes used to describe the care offered to the patient in an attempt to control or reduce the pattern of future disease.

4.2 Caries control (and lesion prevention)

4.2.1 Categorizing caries activity and risk status

On the basis of the history and examination, the patient may be allocated to one of the following in terms of caries activity/risk status:

- **⚠** *Caries inactive/caries controlled/low risk:* no active lesions and no history of recurrent active restorations in the past 2 to 3 years. A level of control (maintenance) is still required to remain in this stable condition.
- **⚠⚠** *Caries active/modifiable risk factors/moderate risk* (plaque control, fluoride, diet): presence of active lesions and a yearly increment of more than two new/progressing/filled lesions in the preceding 2 to 3 years. Caries control may be achieved by changing/modifying risk factors.
- **⚠⚠⚠** *Caries active/unmodifiable or unidentifiable risk factors/high risk* (dry mouth, medications): this category will always be high risk, although it may still be possible to control caries by optimal moderation of such risk factors. Presence of active lesions and a yearly increment of more than two new/progressing/filled lesions in the preceding 2 years.

The aim is to help the patient to change their risk factors so that, at recall, the caries activity status may be deemed to have changed because there are no new active lesions and/or lesions previously judged to be active are now deemed to be arrested. The correlation between current risk status of the patient and the presence of active lesions (and their stage of progress—a *caries risk matrix*) can lead to an assessment being made by the oral healthcare team, in conjunction with the patient, of their likelihood of suffering from new disease in the future. Table 4.1 shows a flowchart of potential care plans depending on active lesion presence and the patient's caries risk. Note that in all cases disease control is paramount in preventing further lesion development, but there are different levels of control that can be offered depending on the activity/risk status—*standard* and *active* care (see Table 4.2).

4.2.2 Standard care (non-operative, preventive therapy): ⚠ low-risk, caries-controlled, disease-inactive patient

The standard care regimen is carried out wholly by the patient on the advice of the suitably trained oral healthcare team dental care professional (dentist, oral health educator, hygienist, or therapist).

Plaque control

Caries lesions form as a result of the metabolic events in the dental plaque biofilm. Thus plaque control is the logical cornerstone of non-operative therapy. Teeth should be brushed with a fluoride-containing toothpaste, as the latter interferes with growth and ecology of the biofilm, and fluoride application retards lesion progression.

The preventive action of tooth brushing can be maximized if the following principles are followed:

- Brushing should start as soon as the first deciduous tooth erupts.
- Brush twice daily, last thing at night, and at one other time each day.
- Discourage rinsing with large amounts of water after brushing—'spit, don't rinse' is the correct advice.
- Evidence exists that using electric rotating/oscillating toothbrushes can be more effective in plaque biofilm removal, but this will be patient dependent.
- Children under 3 years of age should use a toothpaste containing no less than 1000 ppm (parts per million) of fluoride.
- Children between 3 and 6 years of age are likely to swallow toothpaste, and this may cause fluorosis. To prevent this they should use only a smear of paste (a pea-sized amount) on the brush head, and should not be allowed to eat or lick toothpaste from the tube.
- Currently it is recommended that over the age of 3 years, family fluoride toothpaste (1350–1500 ppm fluoride) should be used.

Table 4.1 A care plan flowchart for caries management showing the interaction of caries susceptibility, presence/absence of lesions, and an emphasis on minimally invasive dentistry for the operative treatment of individual lesions with suitable recall intervals

Identify (Chapter 2) Caries susceptibility	Active lesions				No/inactive (arrested) lesions	
	Cavitated (irreversible)	Non-cavitated (reversible)				
	High/low caries risk 3, 4 (mICDAS)	High risk 0, 1, 2	Low risk 0, 1, 2	High risk	Low risk	
Control (prevent) (Chapter 4) Preventive care and patient motivation	**SC + active care plus:** Pit and fissure sealants Patient motivation	**SC + active care:** Remin Fluoride CPP-ACP PMTC Patient motivation	**SC + active care:** Remin Fluoride CPP-ACP PMTC	**SC + active care:** Fluoride CPP-ACP PMTC Patient motivation	**SC + maintenance** Oral hygiene Diet control Fluoride toothpaste	
Restore (Chapters 5 and 8)	Transitional restorations: GIC Long-term direct restorations: GIC/composite/amalgam	Preventive resin restorations	–	–	–	
Recall (Chapter 9)	2–6 months	3–6 months	6 months	3–6 months	12–18 months	

The column on the left indicates where in this book those topics are discussed in more detail. See Table 4.2 for explanations of standard care and active care regimens.

CPP-ACP, casein phosphopeptide–amorphous calcium phosphate; PMTC, professional mechanical tooth cleaning; SC, standard care.

First published in the *Journal of Minimum Intervention Dentistry* 2009; 2: 103–24. Reproduced here with permission.

Table 4.2 Features of preventive care regimens, standard and active care, to control caries and prevent lesions from developing or progressing

Standard care (patient-led, non-operative) ⚠ Inactive/controlled, low-risk patient	Active care (dentist-led, operative/non-operative) ⚠ Active/uncontrolled, high-risk patient
Plaque control (toothbrush and toothpaste, flossing) Use of **fluoride** (toothpaste, water) **Dietary** modification **Continued patient motivation** paramount to prevent onset of disease	**STANDARD CARE +:** **Decontamination** procedures (PMTC, transitional restorations, chlorhexidine) **Remineralization** procedures: • Fluoride (high-concentration toothpaste, mouthwashes, topical varnishes) • Remineralizing pastes/solutions (e.g. CPP-ACP, bioactive glasses) **Managing hyposalivation** (medications, saliva substitutes) **Fissure sealant restorations**

- Children need to be helped and supervised by an adult when brushing.

- The occlusal surface of erupting molars should be individually brushed with the brush placed at right angles to the arch.

- Dependent adults should be helped with tooth cleaning.

Oral hygiene instruction (OHI) should be general to the whole mouth, and site-specific to the particular lesion. The patient should be aware of the problem areas, seeing these in their mouth (via mirrors/images from intra-oral cameras) and/or on a radiograph (with an explanation at a suitable level provided). The following may be helpful with regard to tooth brushing:

- The patient should bring their brush and toothpaste to each appointment they attend.

- Check the toothpaste for fluoride content and the brush head quality to ensure it is not worn.

- Disclose the mouth with a suitable plaque-staining dye so that this can be clearly seen by the patient.

- Assess whether the patient (or parent/carer) can remove the plaque or whether the technique/brush should be altered. For example, arthritic patients may not be able to manipulate the normal handle of a toothbrush, so silicone impression material or cold-cure acrylic may be used to thicken the grip to aid manual dexterity. Rotating/oscillating electric toothbrushes may also be recommended.

- Is thorough brushing in the surgery causing gingival bleeding? If so, does the patient realize that this indicates gingivitis caused by dental plaque?

- If active lesions are present, is the patient aware of where they are and able to remove disclosed plaque from them?

Where active proximal lesions are present, either in the enamel or on the root surface, an interdental cleaning aid will be needed. In young patients, lesions are best cleaned with floss, whereas interdental brushes are preferred for cleaning larger interdental spaces following gingival recession. The following may be helpful with regard to interdental cleaning:

- Advice given must be site-specific.

- Examining the tape or brush after use may show the plaque that has been removed, and this can be a useful motivating factor.

- A special holder for the floss or brush may help the patient.

- Super-floss may be used to clean around bridge pontics or crown margins.

- If the gingivae bleed, the relevance of this should be explained to the patient. If bleeding persists for days after effective cleaning is instituted, this may indicate a cavity or plaque-retentive feature is present that is preventing the patient from removing the plaque. A restoration may be needed to restore tooth integrity to allow the surface to be cleaned.

Use of fluoride

Fluoride delays lesion progression by being incorporated physico-chemically into the hydroxyapatite lattice structure and by inhibiting carbohydrate metabolism within the plaque bacteria (enolase and phosphoenolpyruvate (PEP)-phosphotransferase system inhibition). Vehicles for fluoride include the following:

- *Water*: to date, approximately 15% of the UK population have access to 1 ppm F– water

- *Toothpaste*: fluoride toothpaste is cheap, requires minimal patient cooperation, and enhances patients' appreciation of their essential role in caries control. See page 54 for advice on fluoride concentration and toothpaste use.

The choice of vehicle is not crucial, but it must be combined with improvement in oral hygiene. It is important that the patient accepts the mode of treatment and complies with advice.

Dietary modification

The evidence that the frequency and amount of sugar consumption are linked to caries is irrefutable. Thus an emphasis on diet in caries control would seem logical. Unfortunately, the evidence that it is possible to modify people's diets is lacking! Since the advent of fluoride, the emphasis in caries control has shifted from diet to oral hygiene in conjunction with a fluoride-containing toothpaste. However, this does not preclude the dental care professional from giving dietary advice to all patients. Reducing the amount and frequency of sugary food intake can reduce dental caries and could help weight control. All health professionals have a responsibility to give advice on diet, in the same way as they have a responsibility to give advice on smoking cessation.

No change in diet should be advised for the caries-inactive/controlled patient, but the dentist/team should make the patient aware of how an adverse change in diet and/or salivary flow could pose a future problem, especially if oral hygiene is poor. All patients should be aware of the link between saliva, sugar, and caries.

All of the aspects of *standard care* for controlling disease and preventing lesions require patient cooperation and motivation. The dental team is the adviser, and the patient is the executor of their own preventive care plan.

4.2.3 Active care: ⚠ high risk/uncontrolled, disease-active patient

This regimen includes all aspects of standard care *plus* those listed in Table 4.2, where the dental team may have to take on some of the treatment as well as an advisory role.

Decontamination procedures

Professional mechanical tooth cleaning (PMTC)

This is carried out by members of the oral healthcare team (dentist, hygienist, therapist) using hand scaler/ultrasonic/air-polishing instrumentation to remove gross calculus deposits, and rotating brushes with prophy paste to debride mechanically particularly thick, tenacious plaque deposits on the tooth surfaces. This will then allow the patient to clean more effectively with their toothbrush while enabling the clinician to examine the tooth surfaces directly.

Transitional (stabilizing) restorations

In some cases (e.g. rampant caries), early stabilizing minimally invasive adhesive restorations (high-viscosity glass ionomer cements (GICs)/resin modified (RM)-GICs; see Chapters 7 and 8) can be placed, not only to strengthen remaining tooth structure but also to remove the carious biomass, which acts as a bacterial reservoir and is impossible to clean effectively with conventional oral hygiene procedures (see Figure 4.1).

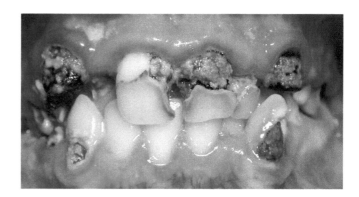

Figure 4.1 An anterior view of a 24-year-old caries-active/uncontrolled, high-risk patient with rampant caries. The large cavitated lesions are covered with a tenacious plaque biofilm. In such patients, transitional (stabilizing) restorations might be necessary to remove the bacterial reservoir and to recontour the smooth tooth/restoration surfaces to facilitate improved oral hygiene procedures.

Q4.1: Look at Figure 4.1. What might be the possible aetiology of this degree of caries attack?

Antimicrobial agents

The present understanding is that dental caries is the result of an imbalanced enrichment of plaque, driven by nutrients that encourage acidogenic and acid-tolerant bacteria (the ecological plaque hypothesis). This may justify the inclusion of some antibacterial agents in a caries prevention regime. These could be incorporated in a toothpaste or mouth rinse. Whatever the delivery method, they should be aimed at:

- minimizing plaque formation
- reducing the growth of specific bacteria
- modifying enzymes that control the production of acid.

Chlorhexidine (CHX) rinses

There is little clinical evidence for the use of chlorhexidine in the medium- to long-term control of caries. CHX (> 0.12%) can affect plaque biofilm adherence and bacterial diversity on a short-term basis, and can be used following oral surgical procedures when normal oral hygiene procedures would be difficult to perform due to pain, risk of post-operative bleeding, and limited access for oral hygiene aids. Due to a high substantivity, its efficacy is related to both concentration and frequency of application. Long-term use may lead to altered taste perception, extrinsic dental staining, and possible mucosal irritation, and is therefore not recommended.

Xylitol

Several studies have shown a significant decrease in *Streptococcus mutans* load after 5 weeks of chewing gum containing xylitol as a sweetener. The minimal effective dose was around 6.5 g per day, divided into at least three chewing periods. Xylitol is safe at the previously mentioned recommended dose, its main side effect—along with other sugar alcohols—being a mild laxative effect.

Remineralization procedures

Fluoride

- High-concentration prescription toothpastes can be beneficial for controlling caries (2800/5000 ppm fluoride) in high-risk patients (multiple lesions, dry mouth). This is because it tips the demineralization/remineralization balance in favour of remineralization, and has the following antimicrobial effects:
  - It impairs glycolysis and metabolic processes in plaque.
  - It inactivates metabolic enzymes.
  - It impairs bacterial membrane permeability to ionic transfer.
  - It inhibits the synthesis of extracellular polymers

- Fluoride mouthwash can be prescribed for patients aged ≥ 8 years, for daily (0.05% NaF)/weekly (0.2% NaF) use. Below 8 years of age, these mouthwashes are not advised because there is a risk of sufficient mouthwash to cause fluorosis in the developing dentition. The rinse should be in addition to twice-daily brushing with toothpaste containing at least 1350 ppm fluoride. Rinses require patient compliance and should be used at a different time to tooth brushing in order to maximize the topical effect, which relates to frequency of availability. The product should be rinsed around the mouth for a timed minute. Be aware that some products are astringent and will be uncomfortable for children and painful for those with a dry mouth and thin, friable intra-oral mucosa. The use of a bland, non-alcoholic mouthwash should be advised. The indications for the use of fluoride mouthwash are:
  - patients over 8 years with high caries activity
  - patients with orthodontic appliances, which inevitably encourage plaque accumulation and predispose to carious lesions
  - patients with a dry mouth (xerostomia)
  - patients with developing root caries. In these patients a weekly concentrated mouthwash may be advised for daily use.

- Professionally applied fluoride varnishes/fluids (e.g. Duraphat, Elmex Fluid) with concentrations of 22 600 ppm F or 2.2% F. Systematic reviews of research have shown that fluoride varnish application by dental care professionals can reduce caries increment in the deciduous dentition by a third, and that in the permanent dentition by nearly half. These are impressive reductions in caries, but the dental professional should be aware of the following:

  - Professional application must be repeated at 3-monthly (high-risk child/adult) to 6-monthly (3 years to teens, adults with dry mouth/active caries) intervals to be effective, and this is inevitably costly.
  - The emphasis switches to the care being provided by the professional rather than by the patient. This is important, as it is essential that the patient is motivated and fully appreciates their own responsibility for maintaining their own oral health. Fluoride is not a panacea for controlling dental disease.
  - The concentration of fluoride is high, and this means that the varnish is potentially toxic to a small child if swallowed. The maximum dose advised for use in the primary dentition is 0.25 ml, and in the mixed dentition is 0.5 ml.
  - The varnish should be applied to isolated, clean, dry teeth. An ideal time to apply varnish is therefore when the teeth are being examined for carious lesions, because in order to detect lesions, the teeth must be isolated, clean, and dry (see Chapter 2). Once the charting is complete, it takes only seconds to apply varnish to fissures, over contact points, cervical margins buccally and lingually, and exposed root surfaces.

Topical remineralizing agents

Much research is being carried out into the development of calcium- and phosphate-rich ionic solutions incorporated, with or without fluoride, into toothpastes, mouth rinses, varnishes, chewing gum, and topical creams, that can act potentially as a reservoir for these mineralizing ions, thereby encouraging surface new mineral deposition. These have the potential to help to combat and prevent caries and dental erosion. An elevated concentration of calcium in plaque biofilm fluid also facilitates a higher build-up of fluoride in this reservoir. In addition, it has been demonstrated that there is a symbiotic relationship between calcium and fluoride. CPP-ACP (casein phosphopeptide–amorphous calcium phosphate) $(Ca_9(PO_4)_6 + H_2O)$ is one such stabilized calcium phosphate system, sold under the trade name Recaldent. ACP has a

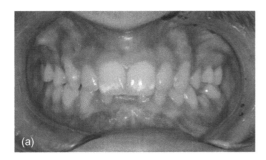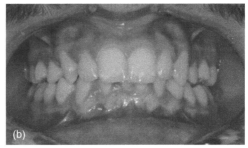

Figure 4.2 **(a)** Patient with chalky, matt fluorotic lesions on the labial surfaces of the upper central incisors (see Chapter 2, Table 2.7). **(b)** The same patient 1 month later, after professional application of topical fluoride/CPP-ACP paste. The lesions are not as clinically evident. (Courtesy of Dr M. Basso.)

Q4.2: How can you distinguish the lesions in Figure 4.2 from white spot carious lesions?

natural predilection to convert to hydroxyapatite (HAP) in wet, ionically favourable environments, and the phosphopeptide chains are thought to help to bind these complexes to the tooth/biofilm surfaces and envelop them, thereby regulating and directing the ultimate precipitation of the HAP where it is needed (i.e. demineralized surfaces). Combinations of CCP-ACP with fluoride have also been developed as pastes and varnishes, and clinical evidence is being gathered as to their overall efficacy in the preventive management of early carious and fluorotic lesions, especially in adults, where the mix of fluoride, calcium, and phosphate ions has a synergistic effect (see Figure 4.2). Current research evidence tends towards a favourable short-term remineralizing effect, but further long-term trials are needed to provide conclusive clinical evidence.

Other calcium- and phosphate-rich formulations include calcium phosphosilicate glass-based dentifrices, functionalized β-tricalcium phosphate, unstabilized amorphous calcium phosphates, nanohydroxyapatite, and calcium sodium phosphosilicate bioactive glass (NovaMin®), which has been combined with sodium fluoride in a toothpaste. Bioactive glass particles produce crystalline hydroxycarbonate apatite in biological aqueous environments over time, encouraging nucleation sites for further remineralization. Recent *in-vitro* studies have shown how these particles may also be used to surface pre-condition white spot lesions using air abrasion, thus aiding new mineral deposition. However, real-life clinical evidence is lacking for many of these formulations, and more medium- and long-term clinical trial data are required.

Managing hyposalivation

As altered saliva quality and production affect up to 20% of the current UK population, and saliva has an important protective role in the oral cavity, the detection of dry mouth (xerostomia) signs and symptoms in general dental practice is of paramount importance. It should be based on the clinical findings from a targeted examination of the quality and quantity of saliva present and the use of a suitably straightforward clinical assessment system, such as the Challacombe Clinical Oral Dryness Scale (see Chapter 2, Table 2.6, and QR code image 2.2). Controlling

caries when the mouth is dry is very difficult. A dry mouth is miserable for the patient, with significant reductions in quality of life indices reported extensively in the literature, and is a concern for the dentist and their oral healthcare team. The long-term management approach for caries control in these high caries risk patients should be as follows:

- Maintain immaculate oral hygiene.
- Prescribe a high fluoride concentration toothpaste (5000 ppm F).
- Prescribe a (non-alcohol-containing) fluoride mouthwash.
- Apply fluoride varnish to existing lesions every 3 months (see previous list).
- Ask the patient to keep a diet sheet and to try to minimize sugar intake.
- Be aware that the patient needs to moisten their mouth frequently, and that plain water is safe.
- Recall the patient every 3 months.
- Saliva production may be stimulated by chewing a xylitol-containing chewing gum, provided there is sufficient salivary gland activity, or pharmacologically.
- In cases of Sjögren's syndrome or post radiotherapy of the head and neck, a saliva substitute may be required, including proprietary dry mouth gels.
- Check that any prescribed antifungal agent does not contain sugar.
- Check with the medical practitioner regarding alternatives to medications that cause hyposalivation (this may be limited, as the medical benefits of the medication will usually outweigh the negative effect of the reduced saliva output).

'Preventive' fissure sealants (FS)

This primary preventive procedure has been included in this section on caries control, as it helps to modify local surface factors that affect the onset and progress of caries and its lesions, namely eradicating caries-susceptible, deep fissures/pits on posterior occlusal surfaces of high-risk patients. There are two types of FS materials:

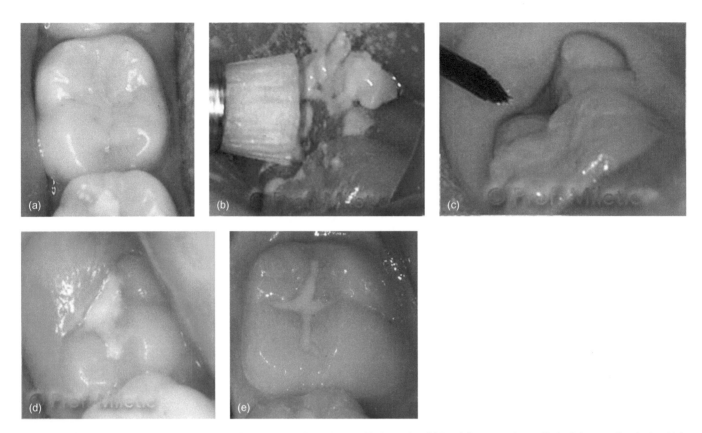

Figure 4.3 **(a)** A glass ionomer fissure sealant on the occlusal surface of a mandibular molar. **(b)** Partially erupted mandibular left second molar in a high caries risk 12-year-old patient with difficult moisture control and access. Occlusal surface is debrided with prophy paste on a rotating bristle brush. **(c)** Ten per cent polyacrylic acid conditioner placed on occlusal surface to remove smear layer. Moisture control is difficult due to the presence of the distal gingival operculum, but was achieved with cotton wool roll isolation (see Chapter 5, Section 5.6). **(d)** The GIC fissure sealant placed (GC Fuji Triage) and **(e)** refurbished 2 years post-eruption in the still caries-free molar. (Figure 4.3 (a) courtesy of the late Dr J. W. McLean; (b)–(e) courtesy of I. Miletic.)

Q4.3:

i. How long would you expect GIC fissure sealants to last? In the patient in Figure 4.3, do you think the FS on the LL7 will need to be replaced indefinitely?

ii. What is the name given to the overlying segment of gingivae on the distal aspect of the occlusal surface on the mandibular molar in Figure 4.3 (d)?

● *Resin-based*: visible light-cured systems based on methacrylate resin composite chemistry (described in Chapter 7). These resins are only lightly filled in order to permit a readily flowable consistency, so creating a void-free infill of deeper fissures. Teeth need to be isolated to obtain effective moisture control, debrided thoroughly, and acid-etched so that the FS is retained micro-mechanically to the enamel surface and light-cured (see Chapter 8, Table 8.2). Care must be taken to ensure the FS is not in direct occlusion, as it will wear or chip readily, with the subsequent risk of increasing plaque accumulation in an uncleansable site.

● *GIC-based:* GICs can be used to bond chemically to the 10% polyacrylic acid-conditioned enamel surface. These materials are more soluble than the resin-based systems, but do leach fluoride ions, which may have a cariostatic effect (see Figure 4.3).

Evidence-based systematic reviews have concluded that there is no clinically significant advantage of one sealant type over another, although it appears that the resin-based sealants show an increased longevity in clinical use when careful application steps are adhered to, and better overall wear resistance. However, in clinical situations where adequate moisture control is difficult to achieve, GIC-based fissure sealants may still be recommended. Both types of FS require careful review and inspection to ensure their long-term integrity. When FS chip or wear away they will need refurbishing, repair, or replacement (see Chapter 9).

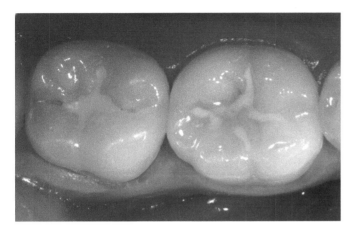

Figure 4.4 Mandibular right first and second molars with aged resin-based fissure sealants. (Courtesy of L. Mackenzie.)

Q4.4: Look at Figure 4.4. What concerns you about the appearance of the aged sealants in the LR6 and LR7?

The detailed clinical procedure of placing a preventive fissure sealant is described in Chapter 8 (Table 8.3). The indications are as follows:

- In high-risk, caries-active adolescents, fissure sealing all erupting molars may be advisable as a primary preventive measure.
- In high-risk young adults where there is evidence of caries on molar teeth which need restoration, other susceptible occlusal fissures may be sealed as a precaution.
- In low-risk, caries-inactive patients with good oral hygiene and minimal/no plaque deposits (checked with disclosing solutions), FS are not generally indicated.
- In young patients with deep fissure patterns, who may otherwise be susceptible due to dietary or other local factors changing (e.g.

mentally/physically disabled, patient undergoing extensive orthodontic treatment, medically compromised).

- Cleaned teeth which can be easily isolated using a rubber dam (see Chapters 5 and 8). Saliva contamination during placement may lead to premature complete loss of the resin-based fissure sealant or leakage at the margins of a partially debonded restoration, which might then lead to active caries. In such clinical scenarios, GIC-based FS may be advised, but with suitable monitoring.

'Therapeutic' fissure sealants

These have been included here as secondary preventive surface treatments for teeth that have undergone early physical damage due to the caries process. Again, most often placed in the pits and fissures of posterior teeth, these sealants are placed with isolation by rubber dam in ideal conditions, after the incipient lesions present have been debrided thoroughly, perhaps remineralized, but not excavated physically. The sealing action of this minimally invasive tooth surface modification, along with suitable maintenance by the patient, will cause the early lesion to become inactive/arrest. There is some ambiguity in this terminology, as the term 'therapeutic fissure sealant' has also been used by some to describe what are known as *preventive resin restorations*, discussed in the following section.

Preventive resin restoration (PRR)/sealant restoration/invasive/ therapeutic fissure sealant

This is placed after the minimally invasive excavation of occlusal caries, up to or just beyond the enamel–dentine junction. In essence, the operator will have undertaken an enamel–dentine 'biopsy' to determine the extent of caries penetration into the tooth. The PRR restores the cavity with a suitable adhesive restorative material (resin composite or GIC) followed by an overlying preventive resin-based fissure sealant which extends on to the unrestored fissures on the remaining debrided and acid-etched sound portion of the occlusal surface, placed as primary prevention for the remaining tooth surface (see Chapter 8, Table 8.3).

4.3 Tooth-wear control (and lesion prevention)

4.3.1 Process

The control and prevention of tooth wear and its lesions are linked intimately with management of the aetiological factors of erosion, attrition, and abrasion discussed in Chapters 1 and 2. The patient's understanding and motivation are vital to the ultimate successful control of tooth wear. The aetiological factors must be identified (by a targeted history and examination) and behaviour modified subsequently (with positive suggestion) in order to remove the causative factor(s). For example, high intake of carbonated drinks/acidic fruit juices over a prolonged period can be adjusted by suggesting that, initially, one in three drinks could be tap water and then, after 1 month, alternate drinks, etc., thereby gradually reducing the primary causative factor.

4.3.2 Lesions

Once structural tooth surface loss has occurred, it cannot be reversed. Early asymptomatic lesions in enamel (or just into dentine) may be left untreated, especially if the causes have been eradicated. The reviewing and recall of patients with pathological tooth wear not requiring immediate operative intervention is discussed in Chapter 9. More extensive tooth loss (accompanied by symptoms including sensitivity, aesthetic considerations, and functional difficulties) can be repaired, depending on the severity, with minimally invasive direct adhesive aesthetic restorations, or with indirect extracoronal restorations (see Figure 4.5). Important factors, including the longevity of the protective restorations placed, and changes in the vertical dimension caused by the tooth surface loss, have to be taken into account in the restorative care plan, details of which are beyond the scope of this book.

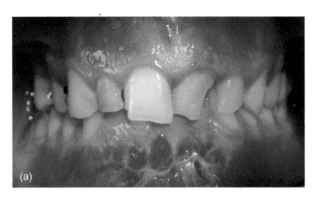
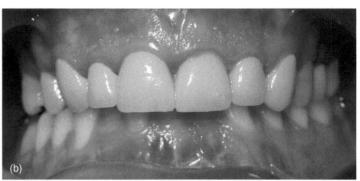

Figure 4.5 **(a)** Preoperative anterior view of a patient with erosion–attrition tooth wear caused by gastro-oesophageal reflux disease. **(b)** Anterior view after treatment with metal-ceramic indirect crowns on UR3 to UL3.

Q4.5: Look at Figure 4.5 and answer the following questions.

i. What might the presenting complaints have been?

ii. The long-term tooth loss has caused a loss in occlusal vertical dimension (see Chapter 5). What clues are present in these images to indicate that this process has occurred?

iii. Do you know what might have caused the scar on the anterior mandibular mucosae?

4.4 Suggested further reading and PubMed keywords

www.ncbi.
nlm.nih.gov/
pubmed/
advanced

QR code image 4.1 Try searching the following keywords on PubMed for relevant further reading. You can access PubMed by scanning the QR code image or at the address .

Keywords

dental remineralizing solutions; CPP-ACP.

 ## 4.5 Answers to self-test questions

Q4.1: Look at Figure 4.1. What might be the possible aetiology of this degree of caries attack?

A: Long-term poor diet and oral hygiene. This appearance is also a presentation of recreational drug-induced caries in young adults—possibly use of methamphetamine or methadone (a viscous, sugary syrup).

Q4.2: How can you distinguish the lesions in Figure 4.2 from white spot carious lesions?

A: The site—discrete white spot lesions are usually found closer to the enamel–dentine junction and sites associated with plaque stagnation. These lesions are present across the incisal third of the labial surface and not associated with plaque.

Q4.3:

i. How long would you expect GIC fissure sealants to last? In the patient in Figure 4.3, do you think the FS on the LL7 will need to be replaced indefinitely?

A: Depending on patient factors, realistically they would probably last for about 2 years or so. This young patient was initially deemed at high caries risk, so the FS was justified. However, over time the preventive oral care undertaken by the patient will hopefully change their risk status. Indeed, this patient maintained a low-risk status and underwent orthodontic treatment. Therefore the GIC FS was not replaced when it finally failed.

ii. What is the name given to the overlying segment of gingivae on the distal aspect of the occlusal surface on the mandibular molar in Figure 4.3 (d)?

A: Gingival operculum.

Q4.4: Look at Figure 4.4. What concerns you about the appearance of the aged sealants in the LR6 and LR7?

A: In the LR6 the FS appears intact, but there is a grey shadow evident. In a high-risk patient one might be concerned whether this was active caries or not. Other signs, symptoms, investigations, and information gleaned from previous notes would be taken into consideration when deciding whether to monitor or to operatively intervene. In the LR7 the FS has chipped at either end of the horizontal fissure. This would be a concern as it would represent a plaque trap that would be difficult for the patient to clean, and it would need to be at least repaired (see Chapter 9).

Q4.5: Look at Figure 4.5 and answer the following questions.

i. What might the presenting complaints have been?

A: Poor appearance, sharp edges of the incisors cutting the tongue, teeth fracturing, sensitivity.

ii. The long-term tooth loss has caused a loss in occlusal vertical dimension (see Chapter 5). What clues are present in these images to indicate that this process has occurred?

A: Note the step up in the line of the attached gingivae of the mandible subjacent to the lower incisors. This is the classic appearance of *dentoalveolar compensation* that has occurred in an attempt to maintain the vertical relationship between the maxillary and mandibular teeth.

iii. Do you know what might have caused the scar on the anterior mandibular mucosae?

A: Post-operative scar after fixation of fractured mandible with a bone plate several years ago.

5

Essentials of minimally invasive operative dentistry

Chapter contents

5.1 The oral healthcare team

All members of the oral healthcare team have a part to play in patient management, and the team is comprised of the lead dentist (plus other colleagues in the dental practice), the dental nurse, hygienist, receptionist, laboratory technician, and possibly a dental therapist. In the UK, registered dental nurses can take further qualifications in teaching, oral health education, and radiography, and can specialize in other aspects of dentistry, including orthodontics, oral surgery, sedation, and special care.

If the dentist wishes to have a second specialist opinion regarding a difficult diagnosis, formulating a care plan or even executing it, they may refer the patient to a specialist dentist working in another practice, or to a hospital-based consultant specialist in restorative dentistry. These specialists have undergone further postgraduate clinical and academic training and gained qualifications enabling them to be registered as specialists with the General Dental Council (GDC) in the UK in their specific trained fields (e.g. endodontics, periodontics, prosthodontics), or have further specialist training in restorative dentistry. The lead dentist will act as a central hub in the coordinating wheel of patient management, possibly outsourcing different aspects of work to relevant specialist colleagues, as spokes of that wheel.

5.2 The dental surgery or 'dental clinic'

This is the clinical environment in which patients are diagnosed and treated. This room has traditionally been known as the 'dental surgery', but a more appropriate modern description might be the 'dental clinic', as much of the more holistic care offered to patients within its four walls will be non-surgical in the first instance. The operator and nurse must work closely together. To be successful, each must build up an understanding of how the other works. The clinic consists of a dental operating chair with an attached or mobile bracket table carrying the rotary instruments and 3-1 air/water syringe (and possibly the light-cure unit and ultrasonic scaler), work surfaces (which should be as clutter-free as possible for good-quality infection control; see later), cupboards for storage, and two sinks, one for normal hand washing and another for decontaminating soiled instruments prior to sterilization. Often the surgery will also house an X-ray unit for taking intra-oral radiographs. Most clinics are designed to accommodate right-handed practitioners, in terms of the location of many of the instruments and controls. In larger clinics there may be space to accommodate a table/desk and comfortable chair where the initial verbal consultation may take place before moving to the dental chair for the clinical examination.

5.2.1 Positioning the dentist, patient, and nurse

All three must be positioned for maximum comfort, visibility, and access while maintaining a healthy posture. Initially, the dentist and patient should be sitting at the same eye level, face to face (see Figure 5.1).

The patient is then reclined in the dental chair into a near horizontal position, and the height of the chair adjusted so that the patient's head is level with the dentist's mid-sternum, whose knees are placed beneath the patient's headrest. The dentist should sit with their back straight and upper arms vertical, with the elbows bent at right angles. Their thighs should be near parallel to the floor and knees bent at right angles, with feet firmly placed flat on the floor (see Figure 5.2). The use of backless saddle chairs can help the clinician to achieve and maintain this posture throughout the working day.

For a right-handed dentist, the nurse should sit to the left of the patient, facing the patient, sitting approximately 10–15 cm higher than the dentist to aid their direct vision into the oral cavity. The nurse's chair may have a foot bar and a swivel back rest that can be moved round to support the nurse when they are assisting the dentist intra-orally. If the patient's head in the dental chair is represented by a clockface with 12 o'clock between the patient's eyes, the dentist can move between 8 o'clock (to view the lower right quadrant with direct vision and the patient slightly more upright in the chair) and 1 o'clock, and the nurse from 1 to 4 o'clock positions (see Figure 5.3). These positions may be reversed for the left-handed operator, assuming that the surgery is designed with this in mind. Some dental chairs are designed so that the nurse's suction and operator's bracket table/mobile cart may be transposed.

The patient can facilitate direct intra-oral vision by moving their head. The dentist should ask and gently guide the movement—a right head turn to view the upper left buccal quadrant, tipping the head down to view the mandibular dentition, and lifting the chin up to view the maxillary dentition.

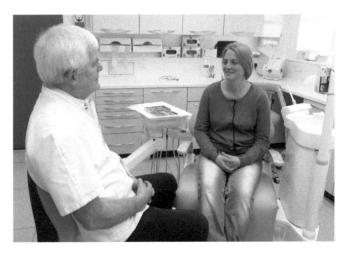

Figure 5.1 Dentist and patient positioning during the consultation. Note how the dentist is sitting slightly in front of the patient and at the same eye level. This positioning enables the patient to feel more comfortable and relaxed.

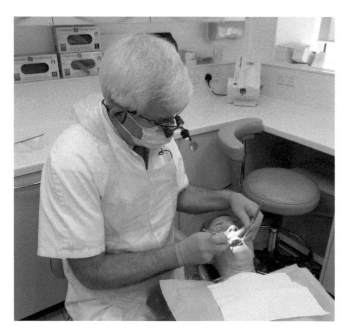

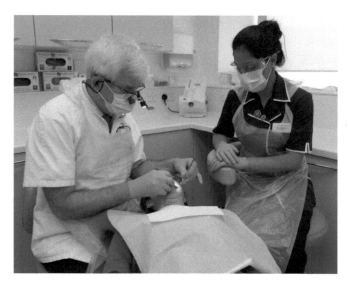

Figure 5.3 The initial positions of the dentist and nurse during the intra-oral examination. See text for details.

Figure 5.2 Dentist operating position with the patient reclined in the dental chair. Note how the operator's elbows are bent at 90° and their back is straight and shoulders relaxed. The dentist is using an LED head-light to help to illuminate his field of view, without shadows.

5.2.2 Lighting

Good-quality illumination is vital in order to work in a patient's mouth. It is usually afforded by the overhead chair light fitted with daylight-simulating light bulbs. These lights may be focused on the patient's face and mouth by correct spatial positioning and alignment (some cast a horizontal dark shadow if incorrectly focused). They should be aligned to cast their beam of light as directly in line with the operator's line of sight as possible (usually offset by only a few degrees), to reduce the shadows cast intra-orally. The intra-oral mirror should be used to direct light specifically to the areas required (e.g. maxillary structures). Light handles must be covered with disposable shields for infection control purposes. An LED headlight can be worn by the operator, focusing the shadowless light in the direction of the dentist's gaze (see Figure 5.2). Care needs to be taken when working with resin composites, as these can be light-cured prematurely by intense LED outputs or the overhead operating light. An orange filter can be used to prevent this from happening when using the LED headlight, or alternatively the operating light may need to be directed away from the oral cavity when placing the resin composite restorative material.

5.2.3 Zoning

For infection control purposes, the dental surgery must be divided into zones for clinical notes/clean instruments and dirty instruments. It is important that these zones are designed with practicality in mind, as thoroughfare between and through them should be kept to a minimum in order to prevent cross-contamination between zones. An example in a hospital setting is shown in Figure 5.4, but variations will obviously be found in different dental practice surgeries. Dirty zones (areas that are likely to become contaminated by direct contact, aerosols, or splatter during treatment procedures) include the following:

- bracket table and handle
- dental handpiece unit, connectors, and switches
- dental chair headrest
- light handles/switch
- chair handle controls
- suction connectors
- spittoon.

These zones must be cleaned and disinfected appropriately between patients. To aid this process, most of the equipment can be covered with clear plastic wrap (cling film) or plastic sleeves, which are removed, the zones cleaned, and plastic wrap replaced between patients.

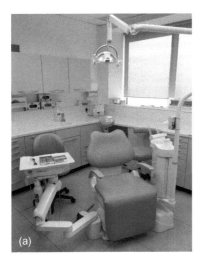 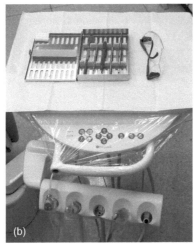 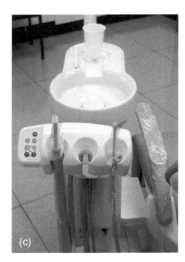

Figure 5.4 The infection control barriers placed when setting up a dental surgery. (a) An overview of the surgery. (b) The bracket table. (c) The spittoon area. Note the use of disposable suction tips and barrier protection on all tubing.

5.3 Infection control/personal protective equipment (PPE)

Current guidelines require the dentist and nurse to be dressed in short-sleeved tunic/uniforms, with no neckties that hang loosely from the neck and no jewellery (except wedding bands). Footwear should cover the tops of the feet. Standard infection control practice against blood-borne, airborne, and other body fluid-borne pathogens is outlined in Table 5.1. With regard to protecting the patient, a disposable neck towel

Table 5.1 Infection control procedures for the oral healthcare team

Infection control precautions	Comments
Hand hygiene	Soap/detergent and running water; alcohol hand gels before donning and after removing gloves
Skin dressings	Cuts, abrasions, and skin conditions protected with waterproof dressings
Sharps handling	Used needles and sharps should be disposed of by the user into rigid sharps containers Only re-sheath needles if using a re-sheathing device/single-handed technique
Personal protective equipment (PPE)	Reusable protective eyewear worn (goggles with side protection or visors over spectacles) if there is a risk of blood/body fluid splashing to the face Single-use surgical face masks provide a physical barrier to splashes to the mouth/face. They do not protect the wearer from aerosol inhalation Respirator-type masks can be used to protect against aerosol inhalation Single-use gloves: natural rubber latex (NRL, non-powdered), nitrile (acrylonitrile)/polychloroprene or Tactylon gloves should be worn (non-allergenic) NRL can result in development of latex hypersensitivity—delayed type IV (contact dermatitis, rhinitis, conjunctivitis up to 48 hours after exposure) or, less commonly, immediate type I (asthma, urticaria, laryngeal oedema, anaphylactic shock usually within 30 minutes after exposure) Single-use plastic aprons to prevent contamination of clothing
Blood/body fluid spillages	Dealt with by using hypochlorite granules and appropriate PPE
Clinical waste handling	Infectious hazardous waste disposed of in yellow clinical waste bags
Instruments	Single-use sharp instruments disposed of in appropriate sharps container. Reusable instruments must undergo decontamination prior to sterilization (see later)

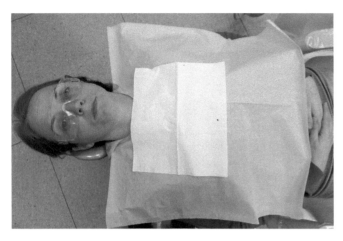

Figure 5.5 Patient in a reclined position wearing eye protection and a disposable bib and neck towel.

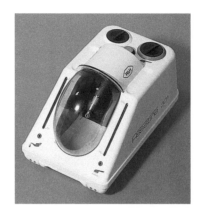

Figure 5.6 An automatic handpiece cleaning unit which is connected to the air supply. The shield at the front is rotated out of the way and the handpiece plugged on to the connector. A detergent is then flushed through the handpiece, followed by oil, both of which come from refillable containers at the back of the unit. This is a quicker and more efficient system than using aerosols.

should be placed over them, and suitable eye protection must be worn by the patient while they are in the reclined position (see Figure 5.5).

5.3.1 Decontamination and sterilization procedures

The days of locating the sterilizing unit in the corner of the surgery are numbered, and in some countries they are long gone (see QR code image 5.1). Separate sterilization facilities for reusable equipment are required (either in a decontamination unit or a segregated area within the surgery) with contaminated entry and clean exit pathways clearly demarcated. This area should be separated into dirty, sterilization, and clean zones. Instruments need to be washed manually and placed in an ultrasonic bath to remove debris. A thermal washer–disinfector is recommended. Dental handpieces require lubrication before and after sterilization, using manual aerosols or an air-driven cleaning/lubricating unit (see Figure 5.6).

Once this decontamination cycle is completed, non-vacuum (downward/gravity displacement bench-top steam) or vacuum bench-top steam sterilization (recommended for wrapped/unwrapped,

QR Code image 5.1 Scan this QR code image with your mobile device to access UK government guidance on decontamination in dental primary care practices (HTM 01-05).

www.gov.uk/
government/
uploads/
system/
uploads/
attachment_
data/
file/170689/
HTM_01-
05_2013.pdf

hollow-lumen items) is required before individual instruments are dried (thus preventing long-term corrosion of carbon steel instruments) and finally bagged in sterile packets and stored in the clean zone. Conventional default settings for most steam sterilizers are 134–137°C held for 3 minutes at a pressure of 2.5 bar. In hospitals, central sterilizing facilities take on this role and soiled instruments are carefully packaged.

5.4 Patient safety and risk management

During operative dental procedures, patient safety is of paramount importance. Accidents will happen, but the risk of these occurring must be minimized or even eradicated at all costs—this is known as *risk management*. In terms of sustaining injury/harm during a dental procedure, the vulnerable areas of the patient include their eyes, airway, and soft tissues. The damage can be caused by inappropriate use/maintenance of sharp instruments, burs, and small instruments, and improper use/handling of dental materials. Table 5.2 outlines the sites, aetiology, and types of injury that might be sustained, and methods to prevent them from occurring.

5.4.1 Management of minor injuries

In all cases of injury, the patient must be informed and the events documented comprehensively in the patient's notes.

- *Eyes*: If debris enters the eyes (of the patient or a member of the dental team), immediate washing in an eye-bath with sterile water is essential, with follow-up medical care if required.
- *Airway*: If an inhalational blockage occurs, stand the patient bent at the hips and firmly slap their back to help to dislodge the object

Table 5.2 A summary of the potential sites/types of patient injury, causes, and methods used by the oral healthcare team to prevent them from occurring

Patient	Aetiology of injury	Type of injury	Prevention
Eyes	Sharp instruments slipping/burs fracturing, fragments of restoration, aerosolized dental materials/body fluids	Laceration, burn, infection	Protective glasses (with side covers) worn when patient is supine
Airway	Small instruments (fractured burs, RCT files), indirect restorations (crowns, inlays), implant components, extracted teeth/fragments	Inhalation or swallowed. Lung infection, blockage of URT airway	Rubber dam; safety chains/floss tied to small instruments; gauze squares placed intra-orally to cover back of throat
Soft tissues (lips, mucosae, tongue)	Caustic dental materials (acid etchant, hypochlorite), sharp instruments (including needles), rotary burs, heat, aggressive retraction of soft tissues, compressed air introduced into open wounds; anaesthetized tissues	Burns, lacerations, grazes, surgical emphysema	Rubber dam placed correctly with sufficient seal; proper use/maintenance of handpieces/burs; single-use needles—*do not bend*. Avoid directing air jets into broken mucosae or exposed root canals

RCT, root canal therapy; URT, upper respiratory tract.

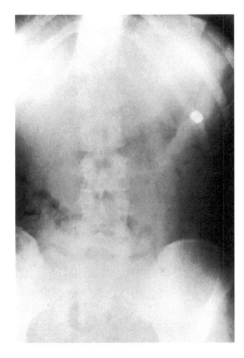

Figure 5.7 Radiograph showing a gold crown in a patient's stomach. (Courtesy of Professor A. H. R. Rowe.)

Q5.1: Can you spot the gold crown in Figure 5.7?

from the oropharynx. Check that the object has not been sucked up the high-volume aspirator (if in use). If the object cannot be accounted for, and the patient is not sure whether they have swallowed it, a chest radiograph will be required to help to localize the foreign object in the bronchi, lungs, oesophagus, or stomach (see Figure 5.7). Follow-up medical attention will be required, especially for the former, as a bronchoscopy may be indicated.

- *Soft tissues*: Haemostasis of cuts and abrasions must be achieved. Cuts to the lips or mucosae may need sutures. Caustic sodium hypochlorite burns (caused by a leaking rubber dam in root canal therapy) may require medical attention and a suitable dressing to promote healing without scarring. Patients with inferior alveolar nerve anaesthesia should be warned about the persistent numbness that will occur for several hours after treatment, and advised to take care to avoid biting/chewing their lower lip or consuming hot food or drink in case they burn themselves.

5.5 Dental aesthetics and shade selection

The advent in the early 1960s and continued development of direct adhesive, tooth-coloured restorative materials have raised patients' expectations with regard to high-quality aesthetic results when it comes to restoring teeth to form and function, especially in the anterior 'aesthetic zone' (UR4–UL4). Indeed, we are now at a stage in minimally invasive conservative dentistry where all operative interventions should be aesthetic in nature. An aesthetically pleasing dental result depends on numerous complex and interlinked factors, including:

- the three-dimensional shape and position of the tooth
- the surface form and finish of the tooth
- the inherent shade of the tooth
- the morphology of the surrounding periodontal and facial tissues
- the occlusal plane and relationship with adjacent/opposing teeth.

The dental materials that can offer shades and characteristics that closely match natural tooth aesthetics are, in descending order:

- dental porcelains (indirect—made by a dental technician in a laboratory from casts poured from dental impressions and finally cemented in/on the tooth)
- dental resin composites (direct—placed at chairside; indirect—made in the laboratory)
- glass ionomer cements (direct—including conventional, resin-modified, and polyacid-modified composites).

5.5.1 Colour perception

The human brain is able to perceive intrinsic physical properties of incident light sensed by the eye. In order to communicate these, colour scales have been devised. One of the earliest was the system from A. H. Munsell, which consisted of three elements—the dominant wavelength (*hue*), the excitation purity (*chroma*), and its luminous reflectance (*value*) (see Table 5.3).

However, the human tooth is heterogeneous, and the pulp, dentine, enamel, their interfaces, and relative thicknesses along with their changing histological structure all play a part in overall perception of the shade by affecting the interaction between incident light and tooth structure. When attempting to mimic the shade of a tooth, the inherent structure of the restorative material and how it affects the physical characteristics of incident light must be considered (i.e. the reflectance, translucency, opacity, and fluorescence). As the Munsell classification does not take these factors into account, another classification was devised by the Commission Internationale de l'Eclairage (CIE)—the CIE L* a* b* colour space. This classification applies the

Table 5.3 The intrinsic physical properties of light perceivable by the human eye according to the Munsell colour space classification

Property of light	Comments
Hue (wavelength)	Wavelength of coloured light translated as its actual colour (e.g. red, green, blue, etc.). Figure 5.8 shows the Vitapan Classical shade guide tabs arranged in the four-lettered groups according to hue: A, more reddish-brown; B, yellow; C, yellow-grey; D, more reddish-grey
Chroma (saturation)	Strength/dominance of the colour (hue). Light or dark shade. Figure 5.8 shows the Classical shade tabs arranged with increasing chroma (1–4) in each of the hue (colour) groups (A–D)
Value (greyness)	Luminosity of the colour (the level of black or white—its *greyness*). Figures 5.9 and 5.10 show the shade tabs arranged in descending order of value. Enamel thickness is the major contributor to the value of a tooth

amount of red, green, and blue colours used. L* measures lightness (0–100, black–white) and CIE a* and b* the relative hue and chroma (a*, levels of red(+)-green(−); b*, levels of yellow(+)-blue(−)). This system permits quantification and calculation of colour numerically, expressed in units that can be related to visual perception and clinical significance. This scale is used in research studies into colour and also the electronic shade guides (see later). The properties of the restorative material that can help to mimic these interactions include the following:

- *Refractive index*: Refraction is the change in direction of light due to it entering a medium of different density. Different materials have

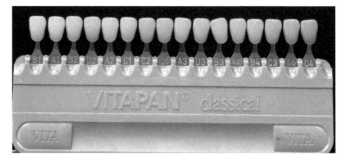

Figure 5.8 The Vitapan Classical shade guide tabs, arranged in four groups, A–D, according to hue (colour) and, within each hue, a range of increasing chroma, 1–4.

Figure 5.9 The Vitapan Classical shade guide tabs arranged in order of value, from high (whiter) to low (darker).

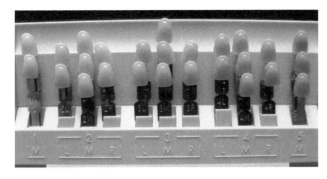

Figure 5.10 The Vitapan 3D-Master shade guide with value graded from 1 to 5 (light to dark), three chroma choices within the value groups 2, 3, and 4, and the individual hue (yellow-red).

different refractive indices. The difference between the refractive indices of two materials determines how opaque or translucent one appears when observed from the other. The opacity of a resin composite depends on the difference between the refractive index of the resin composite material and the refractive index of air (refractive index of vacuum/air, 1.0; water, 1.33; enamel, 1.63; dentine, 1.54; cementum, 1.58).

- *Scattering coefficient*: Scattering is the loss of light due to the reversal of its direction. The scattering coefficient varies with the wavelength of the light and the nature of the colourant layer of a composite. A composite with a higher refractive index (dependent on the polymer matrix, size/type/amount of filler particles, and aluminium/zirconium/titanium oxide opacifiers present) will appear more opaque.

- *Absorption coefficient*: Absorption is the taking up of light by a material. The absorption coefficient also depends on the wavelength of light and the nature of the colourant layer of the resin composite. The higher the absorption coefficient, the more opaque and intensely coloured the resin composite will appear.

When restoring a tooth with a direct resin composite, it is advisable to use incremental layering techniques in order to copy these variations that occur within the tooth. In a young tooth, the thicker enamel will affect the value and hue, with the dentine contributing to the chromatic aspect of its shade. As the tooth ages and the enamel thins, the dentine and pulp will have more of an influence on the hue, with enamel contributing primarily to the value of the final shade. The enamel–dentine junction (EDJ) contributes to the fluorescent characteristics (which can be added in a layering technique using coloured tints and stains). The quality of the surface finish and form will affect the reflectivity of incident light; using a flowable, translucent low filler particle content resin composite will assist in producing a smooth, blemish-free surface after careful polishing (see later). Some manufacturers provide their own

shade guide with their layering resin composite system to simplify the choice of dentine and enamel shades, often calibrated to the Vitapan Classical system.

5.5.2 Clinical tips for shade selection

- Avoid brightly coloured neck towels. It is helpful to use a light blue neck cloth. Select the shade before placing rubber dam, as teeth become lighter as they dry out.

- Ask the patient to remove bright lipstick or other obstacles, such as hoods or hats, which may affect incident light/shadows.

- Schedule aesthetic restoration appointments early in the morning if at all possible, to avoid eye fatigue.

- The light source should be diffuse, not direct. Use natural daylight where possible. Try to avoid conventional fluorescent light sources.

- Fan the shade guide past the patient's mouth and pick the closest tab. Do not stare. Rest your eyes occasionally. After you have selected the hue, squinting/half-closing your eyes will aid the determination of the value.

- Cold sterilize shade guides to prevent damaging them.

- Shade taking should be carried out after prophylaxis but before tooth isolation and preparation, since dehydration can lighten the natural tooth shade as light is reflected from pore spaces within the enamel as it dries out.

- Select the body shade by examining the centre portion of the tooth (see Figure 5.11). Check with the mouth open and closed (lips parted) for anterior dentition.

- Choose the resin composite shade that most closely approximates the centre portion of the shade guide (see Figure 5.11). Custom-made resin composite shade tabs can be constructed from the specific brand of material used by the dentist. Using glass slabs, various thicknesses of each shade of resin composite can be photo-cured and labelled, and used subsequently for clinical shade selection.

- Place directly and cure the chosen shade of resin composite on the tooth surface to be restored, using the correct thickness of material (see Figure 5.11). No etch or bond is required. The patient can use a face mirror to help them to check and agree to the shade of material selected.

As well as the visual shade guides depicted in Figures 5.8, 5.9, and 5.10, there are electronic shade detectors which shine an incident beam of light on to the relevant tooth and then numerically analyse the reflected light. Care has to be taken when assessing particularly translucent incisal edges, as these instruments can misreport the translucency as a greyer overall shade as a significant proportion of the light passes through the tooth rather than being reflected back.

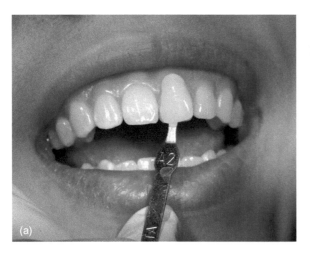
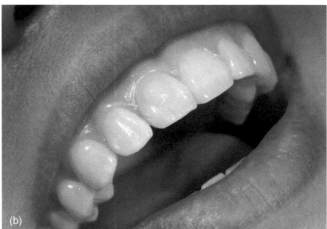

Figure 5.11 Shade assessment of UR1 using a shade tab (left image) to assess the shade from the body of the tab and tooth, and then placing the resin composite on the unetched labial surface of the tooth to make the final assessment, ensuring that the tooth is not dehydrated.

5.6 Moisture control

This is the ability to regulate the fluid environment within the oral cavity and around the individual teeth that is being operated on. Fluids include water, saliva, gingival exudate, and blood.

5.6.1 Why?

Moisture control is required:

- to permit proper placement of all restorations—excessive fluids have a detrimental effect on the adhesion and/or physical properties of all direct plastic restorations, but especially those that rely on adhesive bonding
- to prevent contamination of the restorative procedure—caries removal, direct pulp capping, root canal therapy, and adhesive bonding
- to improve patient comfort—removing accumulated fluids produced by dental handpieces, 3-1 syringes, and salivary flow.

5.6.2 Techniques

- *Aspiration*: Fluids can be evacuated with a single-use saliva ejector by the nurse, the dentist, or even the patient (see Figure 5.12). Plastic tips can be bent into a curved shape to adapt the contours of the lips and oral cavity, thereby accessing the buccal or lingual sulci while simultaneously retracting these tissues.
- *Cotton wool rolls (cellulose pads)*: Used to absorb fluids and retract the lips or cheeks. Placed over salivary duct orifices, upper buccal sulci (parotid ducts), and lingual sulci (submandibular and sublingual ducts; see Figures 5.12 and 5.13). Cotton wool rolls should be rotated into the buccal, labial, or lingual sulci to aid their retention. If still dry at the end of treatment, moisten them with a few drops of water from the 3-1 syringe to facilitate their removal and avoid them sticking to the mucosa.

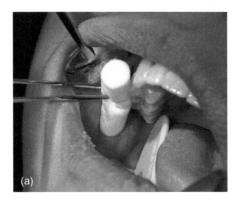
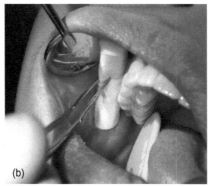
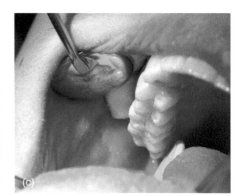

Figure 5.12 Series of images showing how to successfully place a cotton wool roll into the maxillary right buccal sulcus. Note the way that it is rotated into position, thereby ensuring that it will stay in place. A blue flanged disposable saliva ejector tip has been placed lingually to help to retract the tongue.

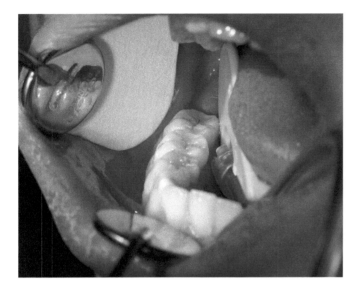

Figure 5.13 A cellulose pad has been used to absorb moisture from the right parotid duct within the maxillary right buccal sulcus.

- *Rubber dam*: A thin latex (or equivalent non-latex—especially important for patients who may be sensitized to latex) perforated sheet that isolates single teeth or groups of teeth, so allowing the best control of moisture. Its advantages and disadvantages are listed

in Table 5.4, and the equipment required to place rubber dam isolation is described in Figures 5.14, 5.15, 5.16, and 5.17.

5.6.3 Rubber dam placement: the practical steps

Figures 5.16 and 5.17 show how a rubber dam can be placed on and then removed from an upper molar using either a wingless (Figure 5.16) or winged clamp (Figure 5.17). Some patients may need local anaesthesia/topical anaesthesia to dull the pain of the clamp on the tooth/periodontium. If a matrix band is required to help to contour the final restoration, the rubber dam clamp may need to be removed as it will get in the way of the circumferential or sectional matrix system (see later). In this situation, the matrix band will take over the role of the clamp in holding the dam in position while the material is packed into place.

For anterior teeth, there is less need to use clamps, as tight contact points can be sufficient to retain the well-adapted dam interdentally, or else a thin strip of rubber dam cut from the peripheral excess/proprietary rubber wedgets can be used by 'flossing' them beyond the contact points. Floss ligatures may also be used. If the contact points are too tight initially for even floss to pass, interdental pre-wedging with a wooden wedge for 5 minutes before placing the dam will usually cause enough tooth movement within its periodontal ligament (and that of the adjacent tooth) to allow the dam to pass between. Careful use of the anterior Ferrier clamp is required so as not to traumatize the gingival margins.

Table 5.4 The advantages and disadvantages of placing and using rubber dam for moisture control

Advantages	Disadvantages
Controlled isolation of the teeth from fluids (reducing adverse effects on bonding/physical properties)	More difficult to communicate with the patient
Reduced bacterial contamination (caries removal, pulp capping, RCT)	Some patients dislike the feeling of claustrophobia (may be reduced by relieving the dam away from the nasal passages)
Patient airway protection from inhalation/swallowing instruments (restorations, burs, endodontic files, wedges); orofacial soft tissue protection from chemical agents (acid-etch gel, dilute hypochlorite solution used in RCT)	Attaching the rubber dam to teeth with clamps can cause pain and some post-operative pain for several hours
Can act as barrier protection from fluid-borne pathogen transfer from patient to dentist	Poorly fitted clamps can cause damage to ceramic crowns (chipping)
Positive psychological experience/improved comfort for some patients. A feeling of detachment/separation from the operation	Care is needed to check medical history for latex allergies for both patient and dentist. Non-latex containing dams are available
Can aid in tissue retraction and so improve direct vision—keeps oral mucosae and tongue separate from the operation field	In inexperienced hands, rubber dam placement can be difficult and time-consuming. However, once it has been mastered, this problem is alleviated
Once in place, rubber dam can speed up the procedure for the dental team	

RCT, root canal therapy.

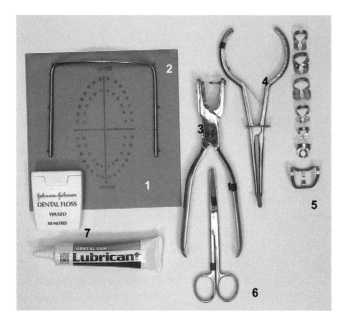

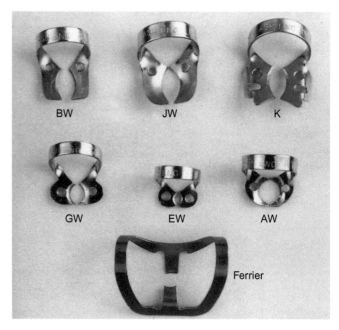

Figure 5.14 Rubber dam equipment comprising:

1. A 15-cm-square dark green rubber sheet (with the position for the perforation holes stamped on using an ink stamp). The rubber resists tearing and grips the tooth surface. Dark colours are used to contrast with the teeth, and torn fragments, often interproximally, can be detected and removed.
2. Metal rubber dam frame holds the free edges away from the face/mouth. The dam is stretched around the tines on the frame itself, keeping it under tension.
3. Rubber dam hole punch, which creates a clean cut perforation of three diameters (corresponding to incisors, premolars, and molars).
4. Rubber dam clamp forceps, used to place, adjust, and remove clamps from teeth.
5. Rubber dam clamps—metal clips that grasp the coronal neck of the tooth holding the dam down. Can be winged or wingless (see Figure 5.15).
6. Scissors to cut excess dam away from the nose and, when removing the dam, interproximally.
7. Waxed dental floss and a water-based dam lubricant—both aid the transition of the dam through tight contact points. Floss can act as a ligature, tying the dam down at the gingival margin.

Figure 5.15 A close-up view of metal rubber dam clamps, consisting of two jaws joined by a curved connecting arm. The two holes accommodate the clamp forceps, which allow the opposing jaws to be separated when placing/removing them over the crown bulbosity. BW, JW, K, and AW clamps are molar patterned (AW is more retentive for partially erupted crowns), GW is used for canines/premolars, and EW is configured for any other smaller tooth. The K clamp is winged—it has two extensions on to which the dam can be placed prior to inserting the dam and clamp together on to the tooth (useful when isolating just one tooth in the arch). The remaining wingless clamps must be first placed on to the teeth, followed by the manual application of the dam over them. The Ferrier clamp is used for retracting gingivae when isolating anterior teeth, working in the cervical area (care is needed not to traumatize the gingivae and cause blood contamination of the field; see Chapter 7).

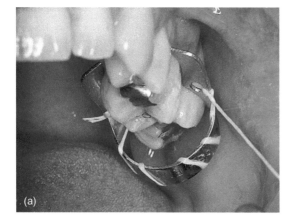

Figure 5.16 **(a)** A wingless JW clamp placed on the UL6. Clamp forceps were used to open the jaws of the clamp sufficiently to allow it to pass over the bulbosity of the crown. Note the floss tied through both clamp holes and coiled around the connector arm. This makes any clamp fragments retrievable if the connector arm fractures under tension when in use. The connector arm is placed distally to prevent the clamp from blocking access to the tooth.

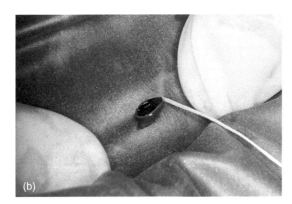

Figure 5.16 **(b)** The dam is stretched gently by the dentist to widen the lubricated perforation, and the free end of the floss is passed through the hole.

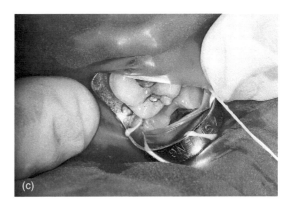

Figure 5.16 **(c)** The dam is stretched over the connector arm first and then over the two clamps embracing the tooth. The nurse can help by keeping the floss taut throughout the procedure.

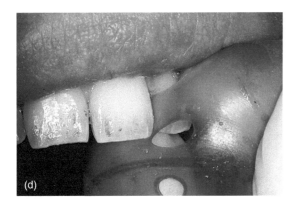

Figure 5.16 **(d)** The dam is then 'knifed' though the contact areas of the remaining teeth to be isolated in the UL quadrant.

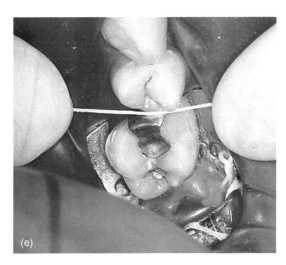

Figure 5.16 **(e)** Floss is used to work the dam down through the mesial contact area of the UL6.

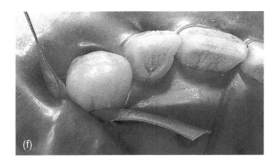

Figure 5.16 **(f)** A strip of dam has been wedged in the distal contact of the UR3 to hold the anterior portion of the dam in place. Sometimes a naturally tight contact may suffice. The dam has yet to be inverted around the cervical margins of the teeth.

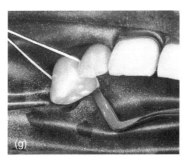

Figure 5.16 **(g)** Alternatively, a floss ligature could be used to the same effect, using a flat plastic instrument to ensure palatal placement apical to the maximum bulbosity of the crown and inverting the dam simultaneously. It will not always be clinically necessary to isolate so many teeth if only working on the UL quadrant.

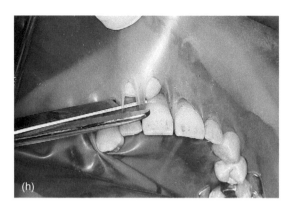

Figure 5.16 **(h)** When removing the dam, it is pulled buccally and cut interdentally using scissors. Note the operator's finger beneath the dam protecting the patient's lip, and the paper towel placed between the dam and the patient's face for comfort (make sure that the nasal airway is not covered by the dam or paper towel). The frame, dam, and clamp are removed together and checked for completeness.

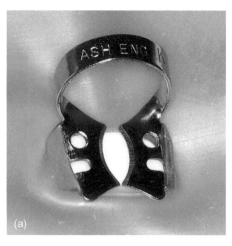

Figure 5.17 **(a)** K clamp (winged molar) with the wings engaged in the lubricated perforation in the dam, outside the mouth.

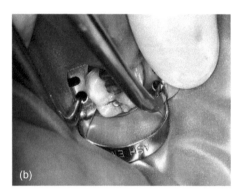

Figure 5.17 **(b)** Clamp and rubber dam being secured to the UL6 as one, using the clamp forceps (note the two pairs of holes to engage the forceps). The nurse can assist the process by gently retracting the loose rubber dam edges to aid vision. Again, the connector arm is placed distal to the tooth being operated upon so as not to block access to instrumentation/visibility.

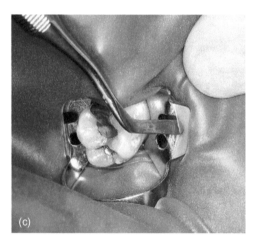

Figure 5.17 **(c)** The dam is disengaged from the wings using a flat plastic instrument, and the contact areas will be flossed to ensure interdental adaptation of the dam.

Q5.2: Can you spot an important clinical omission in Figure 5.17?

5.7 Magnification

Visual magnification aiding clinical examination/operating can be achieved using *magnifiers* or *dental loupes*. A selection of these are shown in Figure 5.18. In terms of optical physics, there are two aspects to consider with regard to their clinical application—the *depth of field (or focus)* and the *field of view (or field width)*.

- *Depth of field (DoF)*: This equates to the distance the operator can move towards or away from the object tooth while keeping the image in clear focus. If this range is limited, procedures become tiring as the operator and patient must always remain at a fixed distance from each other with minimal leeway of movement of either person before the view becomes blurred. For a given magnification, the DoF depends on the f-number of the lens (aperture diameter); ↑ f-number (↓ aperture) leads to an ↑ DoF.

- *Field of view (FoV)*: The angular extent of the observable image viewed through fixed-magnification loupes. Normal unaided human binocular vision (with depth perception) permits 140° FoV. With increasing magnification, this is greatly reduced—for example, 3× magnification with loupes may only permit a clear, sharp view of the object tooth and one either side (depending on the precise optics of the loupes). This can make the introduction of dental instruments into the operating field difficult, and will require the dentist to look away from the loupes' view to do this.

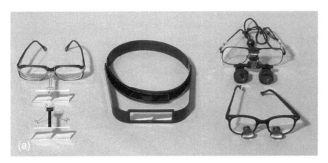
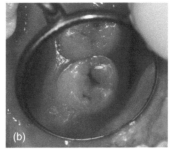
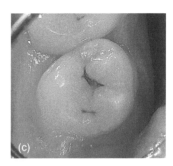

Figure 5.18 (a) A selection of magnification loupes. The first three are the cheapest and have the simplest optics, clipping on to existing spectacles/safety glasses or being secured with a head loop. The two on the right are more expensive. The top right pair have interchangeable lens blocks, and due to their weight require a head cord for retention. Those on the bottom right have the dentist's fixed interpupillary distance built in, as the lenses are cemented through the prescription/safety spectacle lenses. As the magnification optics are closer to the eye, this results in a greater field width and depth of field, but at increased expense. **(b)** The clinical view of an inadequately lit maxillary premolar examined without any magnification. **(c)** The same tooth now lit effectively using an LED head-mounted light along with 2× magnification. More detail can be observed regarding the state of the mesio-distal fissure. ((b) and (c) Courtesy of L. Mackenzie.)

For general dentistry, 2–3× magnification is usually satisfactory, but for endodontics, 4–5× magnification can be used to help to detect root canal orifices and fine root canals. Good visual discrimination in dental procedures requires good depth perception, which in turn requires binocular function. To get the most benefit from the increased magnification, good-quality illumination is also vital. Modern magnification systems often can be fitted with LED lights that are integrated on the frame above the lenses and can be focused on the same focal plane as the lenses. Orange light filters should be used to prevent premature light curing of resin-based materials.

It is the authors' opinion that using magnification to aid the execution of most intra-oral dental procedures is an essential prerequisite for practising high-quality minimally invasive operative dentistry. It is important that the skill of using loupes is learned early on in the clinical skills laboratory, and then transferred to the clinical situation. The physical adjustments made by the operator when using loupes involve practice with a learning curve.

5.8 Instruments used in operative dentistry

Instruments are used to examine, clean, cut, and restore teeth. The main types of cutting instruments are either hand-held or rotary instruments driven in a handpiece. Other equipment includes fibre-optic lights for illumination, light-curing systems used for polymerization of resin-based materials, new instruments for tooth cutting/caries removal, and ultrasonic scalers (see Table 5.5). These instruments may be reused

Table 5.5 Tooth-cutting/caries removal technologies, the substrates acted on, and the mechanism of action

Mechanism	Substrate affected	Tooth-cutting technology
Mechanical, rotary	Sound or carious enamel and dentine	SS, CS, diamond, TC, ceramic, and plastic burs*
Mechanical, non-rotary	Sound or carious enamel and dentine	Hand instruments (excavators, chisels), air abrasion (alumina/bioactive glass), air polishing (sodium bicarbonate/bioactive glass /beta-TCP)†, ultrasonics, sono-abrasion
Chemo-mechanical	Carious dentine	Caridex (of historical value, not available now for clinical use), Carisolv™ gel (amino acid based), Papacarie® gel (papain based), experimental pepsin-based solutions/gels
Photo-ablation	Sound or carious enamel and dentine	Lasers
Others	Bacteria	Photoactive disinfection (PAD), ozone

*Works only on carious dentine.

†Primarily used for stain removal.

SS, stainless steel; CS, carbon steel; TC, tungsten carbide.

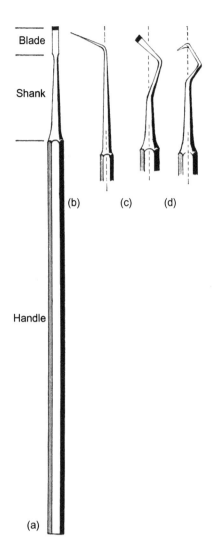

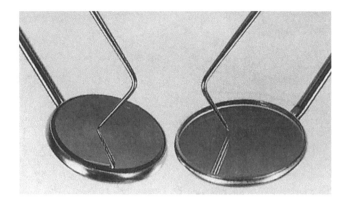

Figure 5.20 Front- and rear-surface mouth mirrors. The left mirror (front-surface) gives a clearer image than the rear-surface 'double' image (right), but is more prone to scratch damage during use and sterilization procedures.

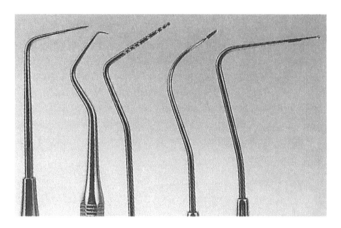

Figure 5.21 A selection of dental probes (from left to right): straight, Briault, Williams, Nabers, and CPITN probes.

Figure 5.19 **(a)** The parts of a hand instrument. **(b)** A straight dental probe with a single bend taking the working tip well away from the handle's long axis, thus aiding direct vision. **(c)** Two bends in a hatchet. **(d)** Three bends in a Briault probe. Medical-grade stainless steel cutting edges can be resharpened using a sharpening stone with oil lubricant (fine edge) or a dry abrasive disc (coarse edge). Tungsten carbide tips should be sent to the manufacturer for resharpening.

Q5.3: In which clinical situations might you use each of the probes shown in Figure 5.21?

after suitable decontamination and sterilization procedures, or else are disposable, single-use items.

5.8.1 Hand instruments

Manufactured from medical-grade stainless or carbon steel (sometimes with tungsten carbide brazed to the cutting edges for increased longevity of sharpness), the majority of hand instruments are designed with a handle, shank, and blade configuration (see Figure 5.19).

Hand instruments can be used for the following purposes:

- Oral examination (mouth mirror, selection of dental probes, pair of tweezers):
  - *Mouth mirrors*: front- or rear-surfaced (see Figure 5.20)

- *Dental explorers/probes*: sharp probes (straight and Briault) are used for checking restoration margins and carious dentine to be excavated within a cavity. Round-ended/blunt periodontal probes are used for periodontal tissue examination and assessing the roughness of enamel/occlusal/smooth surfaces during caries lesion detection/examination (see Figure 5.21)
  - *Locking tweezers*: to place/remove cotton wool rolls, and remove larger pieces of intra-oral debris.
- With the advent of modern infection control guidelines, disposable examination instruments are now manufactured from plastic to allow single use only (see Figure 5.22).
- Periodontal scaling: a selection of *hand-held scalers* (see Figure 5.23) to remove supra- and subgingival calculus deposits.
- Caries removal (excavators, chisels/hatchets/hoes):

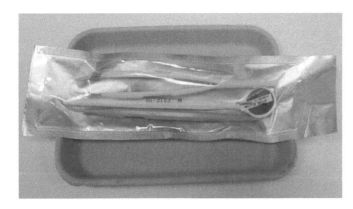

Figure 5.22 Disposable, single-use, plastic examination instruments—mirror, probe, and tweezers—in their sterile packaging.

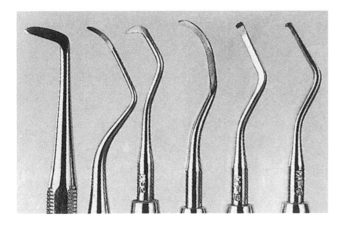

Figure 5.23 A selection of hand-held periodontal scalers (blade and shank visible). Note the angulation of the heads and the extent to which the cutting blades are offset from the long axis of the handle.

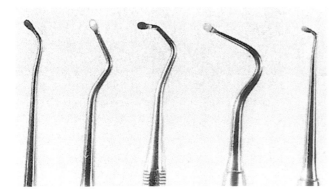

Figure 5.24 A selection of hand excavators (blade and shank visible). Note the different ovoid blade sizes and offset angulations.

Q5.4: What are the advantages of having angulations between the working head and shank of the instruments pictured in Figure 5.24?

- *Excavators*: instruments with a discoid/ovoid blade sharpened to a cutting edge are used to remove caries and soft temporary restorations. Can also be used to shape plastic restorative materials (see Figure 5.24)
- *Chisels, hatchets and hoes*: used to remove unsupported enamel/bevel cavity margins (especially where access for rotary instruments is limited). Hatchets and hoes are similar to chisels in having a straight bevelled cutting edge, and are always angled or contra-angled. They differ from one another in that the cutting edge of the hatchet is in the plane of the shank (like an axe), whereas the cutting edge of the hoe lies in an axis at right angles to this plane (as in a gardener's hoe; see Figure 5.25).
- Handling restorative materials (flat plastics, condensers (pluggers), carvers):
  - *Flat plastic instruments*: used for conveying, placing, and shaping plastic materials that do not require heavy pressure. Usually made of stainless steel, but for composite placement, Teflon-coated or titanium nitride-coated blades confer a useful non-stick property (see Figure 5.26)
  - *Condensers (pluggers)*: smooth surface instruments for packing plastic restorative materials into cavities under pressure (eliminating voids) (see Figure 5.26)
  - *Carving instruments*: sharp/semi-sharp blades that carve the shape/contour of the final restoration by a cutting/scraping action. Different patterns exist (e.g. Ward's, Half-Hollenback) (see Figure 5.26).

5.8.2 Rotary instruments

Dental burs, stones, and cutting and polishing discs are small instruments ('drill bits') gripped firmly by a chuck in a handpiece ('dental drill') powered directly by compressed air, the *air turbine*, or by a separate motor that is either air or electrically driven, the *low-speed* handpieces.

- *Air-turbine ('high-speed') handpieces*: clockwise rotary speeds between 250 000 and 500 000 revolutions per minute (rpm) but relatively low torque, achieved by a small air-driven turbine or rotor mounted in bearings in the head of a contra-angled handpiece. Burs

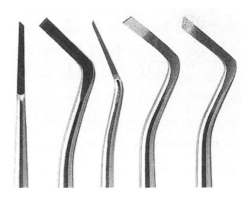

Figure 5.25 A selection of straight and angled chisels (from left to right): straight, hatchet, hoe, and a pair of double-ended gingival margin trimmers.

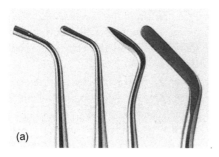
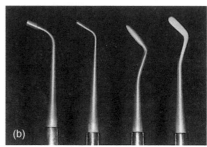

(a)　(b)

Figure 5.26 Stainless steel and titanium nitride-coated (non-stick, gold-coloured) instruments for conveying, placing, and shaping composite materials. Left to right in both images: Guy's pattern condenser (plugger), burnisher (to adapt material to cavity margins), carving instrument (Half-Hollenback pattern), and flat plastic.

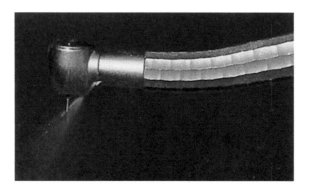

Figure 5.27 Air-turbine handpiece in operation showing the directed water spray over the tip of the bur and the fibre-optic light.

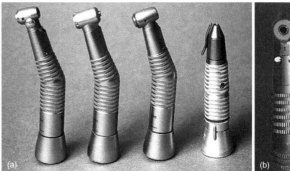
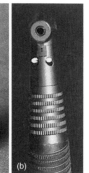

(a)　(b)

Figure 5.28 A selection of low-speed handpieces. From the left:

1:1 contra-angled handpiece used for most procedures. Latch-grip burs are used. Commonly identified with a blue-coloured band on the shank of the handpiece and a blue dot on the head. Speed in the range 400–40 000 rpm.

1:4 speed-increasing handpiece. Friction-grip burs. Operates at 16 000–160 000 rpm. Commonly identified with a red band. Useful for finishing cavity preparations and also finishing restorations.

7:1 speed-reducing handpiece. Latch-grip burs. Used for drilling pin holes and other procedures where slow speed is indicated. Operates at 550–5500 rpm and is commonly identified with a green band.

Straight handpiece that takes straight burs (may be modified to take latch-grip burs). A 1:1 handpiece is identified with a blue band; speed-reducing is identified with a green band. Used to trim temporary restorations and other similar procedures. Usually used outside the mouth.

A fibre-optic light system built into the head of a contra-angled low-speed handpiece.

are held via a friction-grip shank, the tip shrouded in water spray and illuminated with a fibre-optic light (optional; see Figures 5.27 and 5.28).

- *Low-speed handpieces*: two-piece system comprising an electric or air-driven motor coupled to a contra-angled or straight handpiece (rotating clockwise or anticlockwise), with water spray and fibre-optic light; it has lower speed but higher torque than the air-turbine handpiece (see Figure 5.28).

- *Dental burs* (see Figures 5.29 and 5.33), *stones* (see Figure 5.30), and *finishing burs/discs* (see Figures 5.31 and 5.32): gripped in handpieces by a quick-release clamping chuck (friction-grip diamond grit/tungsten carbide (TC) cutting blades for air-turbine handpieces; latch-grip carbon steel/diamond grit/TC/plastic cutting blades for low-speed handpieces).

5.8.3 Using hand/rotary instruments: clinical tips

- Rotary instruments 'cut' hard dental tissues by chipping and smashing mechanically at dental hard tissue ultrastructure. Therefore the resulting prepared surface is often damaged at the microscopic level (see Figure 5.34). This effect has implications when considering the suitability of these surfaces for adhesive bonding (see later).

- Rotary instruments generate heat at the cutting interface (dissipated by the water spray from both high- and low-speed handpieces), as well as vibration, pressure, and noise (all of which are unpleasant for patients). They provide a reduced tactile feel compared with hand instruments, and therefore cutting is guided visually. As a general

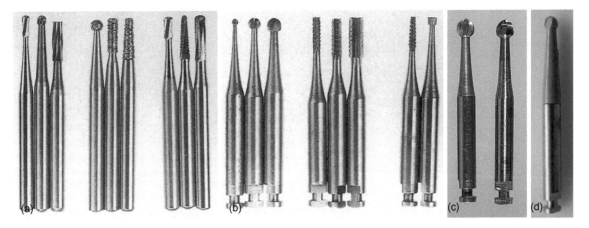

Figure 5.29 A series of eight sets of burs (first three sets, friction-grip for the air turbine; next five sets, latch-grip for the low-speed handpiece).

(a) Friction-grip: tungsten carbide (TC) ×3, diamond grit (round, straight, tapered) and metal-cutting (serrated cross-cut TC blade) burs. TC and diamond used for cutting sound enamel and dentine, removing existing restorations. Diamond burs can be used to cut ceramic.

(b,c) Latch-grip, carbon steel: three sizes round (rose-head), three sizes straight cross-cut fissure, tapered cross-cut fissure, and inverted cone burs (now rarely used clinically). Burs numbered according to size/diameter of cutting head. Carbon steel heads used for cutting carious dentine but blunt quickly, corrode if not dried after sterilization, now often used as a single-use bur.

Similar size carbon steel and TC rose-head burs compared. The TC head is a slightly different shape and is attached to the steel shank. Greater longevity and autoclavable.

Developments have included the latch-grip, rose-head pattern PKK (polyketone-ketone) plastic bur **(d)**, for 'self-limiting' carious dentine removal, single-use.

Q5.5: What might be the advantages and disadvantages of single-use, disposable burs?

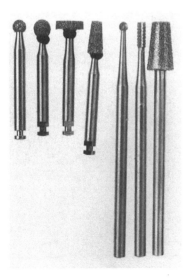

Figure 5.30 A selection of four dental stones mounted on latch-grip short shanks (abrasive carborundum green stones) and three long-shank instruments. Far right is a diamond-coated cone-shaped bur for use in the dental laboratory or rarely at the chairside, for coarse adjustment of indirect restorations and appliances, used at medium speed in a straight handpiece.

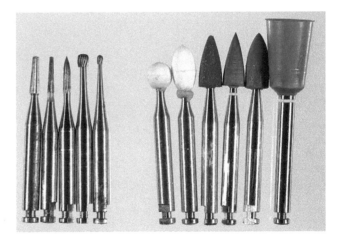

Figure 5.31 Finishing burs, stones, and points for dental amalgam. From the left: five plain-cut latch-grip steel finishing burs, two mounted white (alundum) stones, three mounted abrasive rubber points from coarse to fine, and a mounted abrasive rubber cup.

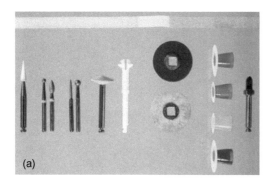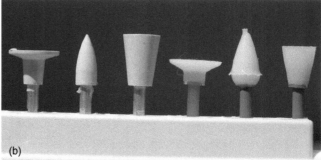

Figure 5.32 (a, b). Resin composite finishing burs/discs. Across the top is a proximal plastic finishing strip with a blank area in the middle to facilitate passage through the contact point between the teeth. On the right portion the abrasive is coarse and on the left it is fine. From the left: a mounted fine white stone, two medium-grit composite finishing diamonds (yellow band), two fine-grit composite finishing diamonds (red band), a mounted abrasive rubber disc, a mandrel for the two abrasive single-sided flexible discs, which are snap-fitted on to the mandrel, and four colour-coded flexible abrasive discs (coarse to fine impregnated grit/diamond) mounted on plastic stubs which fit the mandrel to the right of the picture. In the right image is a series of rubber/resin discs, points, and cups impregnated with silica grit, enabling the finishing of resin composite and glass ionomer cement restorations.

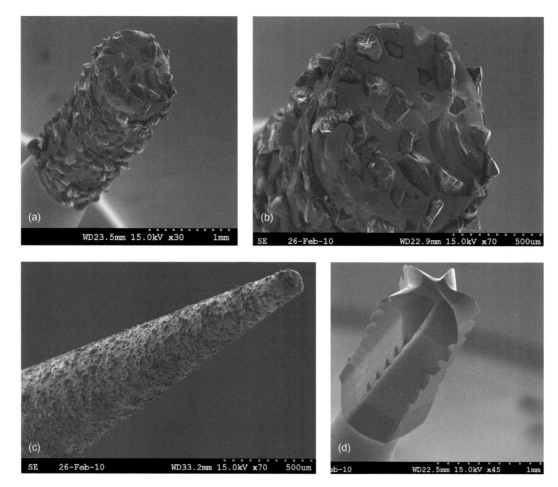

Figure 5.33 (a) Scanning electron micrograph (×30) of a coarse-grit diamond bur. **(b)** The same bur as in **(a)** at 70× magnification showing the random, irregular shapes of the diamond grit. **(c)** 70× magnification of the yellow stripe diamond composite finishing bur with a much smaller grit particle size than the bur in **(a)** or **(b)**. **(d)** 45× magnification of a tungsten carbide Beaver bur used for cutting amalgam and gold. Note the sharp notches cut into each flute.

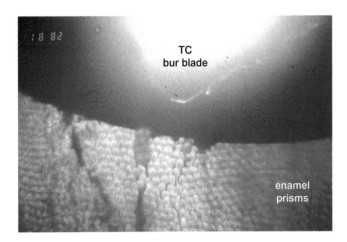

Figure 5.34 Cracks/clefts /cleaving of prisms (horseshoe-shaped structures) after enamel has been cut using a tungsten carbide (TC) bur in an air-turbine handpiece. This inherent damage is unavoidable clinically, but can be minimized by using only gentle pressure when operating, copious water spray, and new, sharp burs in a handpiece with sound bearings, allowing vibration-free rotation. The surface and subsurface damage will have implications for adhesive bonding, as the shrinkage stresses of adhesive materials exerted on these weakened prisms may open up the cracks, further leading to cohesive failure (field width 200 μm).

rule, hard materials (sound enamel, cast metals, and restorations) are cut more efficiently at high speeds and less pressure, whereas softer material (caries) is removed more efficiently at lower speeds and higher torque.

- Water spray ejected from tiny nozzles built into the handpieces should be directed to the tip of the rotating bur head (see Figure 5.27). This cools the tooth surface as it is cut, so preventing excessive frictional heat generation from having a deleterious effect on the pulp. It also helps to flush away debris from the cut tooth surface and the bur head itself. The dental nurse should endeavour to keep the mouth mirror free from spray during rotary instrument use, using the 3-1 air/water syringe and aspiration.

- Some handpieces, when coupled to the main dental unit enabled with fibre optics, have the ability to transmit the fibre-optic light from the head of the handpiece directly on to the bur head (see Figure 5.28). This can greatly improve direct vision.

- Air-turbine, rotary burs produce less vibration and pressure. Latch-grip burs have the potential to vibrate.

- The cutting action of rotary (and hand) instrumentation causes a *smear layer* to be formed on cut hard tissue surfaces (usually < 100 μm thick). This is a tenacious layer of organic, inorganic, and bacterial debris which is either removed or incorporated in a modified form into the bond when placing an adhesive restoration (see Chapter 7, Section 7.2.4).

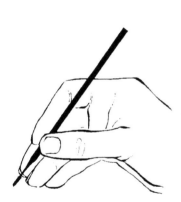
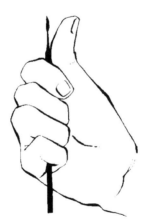
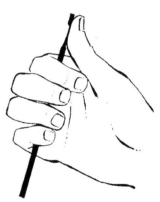

Figure 5.35 From left to right: pen (most common, most control for fine movement), palm, and finger grip of hand instruments. The latter two have a more limited use for more forceful movements in the maxillary arch. Instrument is held between the thumb (for support) and forefinger with the handle across the palm, clasped by the remaining fingers.

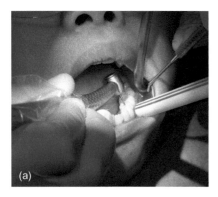 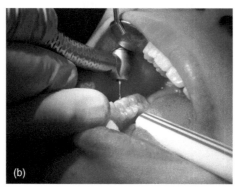 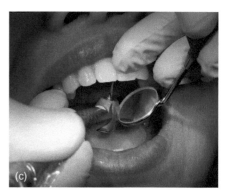

Figure 5.36 Examples of finger rests used by a right-handed dentist while operating a dental handpiece. On the left is a finger rest on the mandibular incisors when operating in the mandibular left quadrant. The middle picture depicts the finger rest on the mandibular right lateral incisor/canine when operating on the mandibular right quadrant. The right image shows a finger rest on the maxillary right canine/premolar region when accessing the maxillary anterior teeth.

- Finger rests: support required for both hand and rotary instrumentation can be achieved by resting the free fingers of the operating hand on a firm structure in the patient's mouth (i.e. adjacent/contralateral/opposing teeth). This provides fine control and reduces the risk of iatrogenic damage, especially if the patient moves suddenly and unexpectedly (see Figures 5.35 and 5.36).

- The free hand is used to hold the mouth mirror to provide indirect vision of the maxillary arch, reflect light intra-orally, and retract soft tissues.

- For the inexperienced operator using rotary instruments (and even some experienced ones!), there is a risk of damaging adjacent sound teeth/restorations (operator-induced, *iatrogenic* collateral damage). As a novice, there may be a case for protecting the adjacent tooth surface with a matrix band when operating proximally, but this then has the disadvantage of interfering with vision.

- With respect to caries removal, burs are not self-limiting, and rely on the operator to distinguish between tissue that requires excavation and that which does not. There has been research into the development of a plastic, single-use bur (see Figure 5.29) which only removes tooth structure that is softer than itself (anything harder and it will blunt during use) and so is more self-limiting. Hand excavators rely on the tactile feedback offered to the operator to distinguish the tissue requiring excavation and permit finer discrimination between the carious dentine zones (infected vs. affected vs. sound; see Chapter 1) than rotary instrumentation.

5.8.4 Dental air abrasion

- Developed in 1945 by R. B. Black, air abrasion is a pseudo-mechanical method for cutting hard dental tissue where the tooth surface is bombarded with high-velocity dry abrasive particles in air, transferring kinetic energy to the tooth surface, which is micro-chipped away.

- Adjustable parameters include the air pressure, powder flow rate, operating distance, type/size/morphology of the abrasive particle, and diameter of the nozzle tip, which all affect the efficacy and rate of cutting.

- Particles approved by the US Food and Drug Administration (FDA) or with CE accreditation for clinical use in the mouth include > 27 μm alumina and bioactive glass powders.

- Useful for minimally invasive operative/reparative dentistry with no heat, vibration, pressure, pain, or noise generated—rapid operator-dependent tissue removal with alumina particles. The extent of surface/subsurface hard tissue damage (cracks/cleft formation) is far less than when using rotary instruments, so making the air-abraded hard surface more suitable for adhesive bonding (see Figure 5.37).

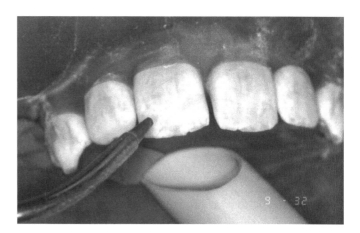

Figure 5.37 An air-abrasion handpiece being used to prepare the labial enamel surfaces of the upper anterior teeth for direct resin composite veneers. Powder used: dry, 27 μm alumina. Note the blue aspirator tip held close to the operating field to vacuum up the spent powder.

Q5.6: What clinical situations may benefit from using air-abrasion tooth preparation?

- Bioactive glass particles can be used for extrinsic stain removal, desensitization of exposed cervical dentine, composite removal, and selective demineralized enamel removal (e.g. preventive resin restorations in high caries risk patients, cleaning residual resin cements after orthodontic bracket removal). Research also indicates a potential use of bioactive glass powders to aid remineralization of white spot lesions.

- New powders are being investigated for self-limiting carious dentine removal and their remineralization potential.

- Multi-chambered air-abrasion units allow a metered flow of different particles (alumina, bioactive glass, sodium bicarbonate) in a shroud of water, reducing the dust generated by the process and permitting instantaneous initiation and termination of the abrasive stream (see Figure 5.38); rubber dam is advisable for patient comfort.

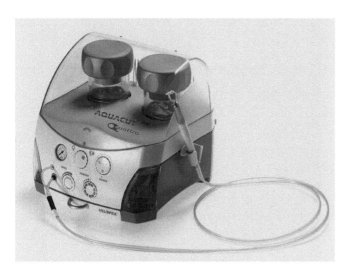

Figure 5.38 An example of a two-chambered dry/wet cutting air-abrasion unit.

5.8.5 Chemo-mechanical methods of caries removal: Carisolv™ gel

- This is a gel-based dentine caries removal system that reacts with carious dentine that has undergone proteolytic breakdown of collagen, causing further collapse of the collagen network for easy final removal with curetting hand instruments or ceramic/plastic burs in a speed-reducing handpiece. This chemistry confers an element of self-limiting caries removal ability.

- Consists of a 0.1% hypochlorite-based alkaline gel (pH 11) with amino acids preventing breakdown of sound collagen fibrils.

- Stainless steel abrasive, non-cutting hand instruments permit carious dentine removal from cavities (see Figure 5.39). The system requires cavitated lesions for direct access to the carious dentine. Ceramic or plastic burs can also be used to aid excavation.

- As excavation is concentrated within caries-infected dentine, patients do not always require local anaesthesia. Gentle hand instrumentation pressure (the same force as normal tooth brushing) contributes to improved patient comfort (see Figure 5.40).

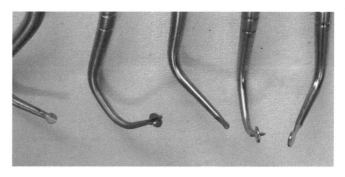

Figure 5.39 A selection of non-cutting, abrasive hand instruments for use with Carisolv™ gel.

5.8.6 Other instrumentation technologies

As can be seen from Table 5.5, there are several clinical methods for cutting teeth and removing caries. Ultrasonic and sonic instrumentation use the principle of probe tip oscillation and micro-cavitation to chip away hard dental tissues. Lasers transfer high energy into the tooth through water, causing photo-ablation of hard tissues. Great control is required by the operator in order to harness this energy effectively, and the effects on the remaining enamel, dentine, and pulp are under investigation in terms of residual strength and adhesive bonding capabilities. Enzymatic (including pepsin-based and papain-based) solutions are being investigated to help further breakdown of collagen in already softened carious dentine in the hope of developing a more self-limiting technique for removing caries-infected dentine alone. Other chemical methods include photo-activated disinfection (PAD)—introducing tolonium chloride into the cavity, which is taken up by the remaining bacteria in the cavity walls and then activated using light of a specific wavelength, so causing cell lysis and death—and ozone (gaseous ozone infused into early lesions, causing bacterial death). These technologies currently suffer from a lack of clinical research to validate them for routine evidence-based clinical use.

It is clear then that minimally invasive operative cutting technologies must aim to preserve as much naturally repairable tooth structure as possible, and at present no perfect instrument exists. Therefore the operator's knowledge of the histology of the dental substrate must be combined with their understanding of adhesion chemistry and the clinical handling of the restorative materials and instruments, if they are to operatively manage caries successfully.

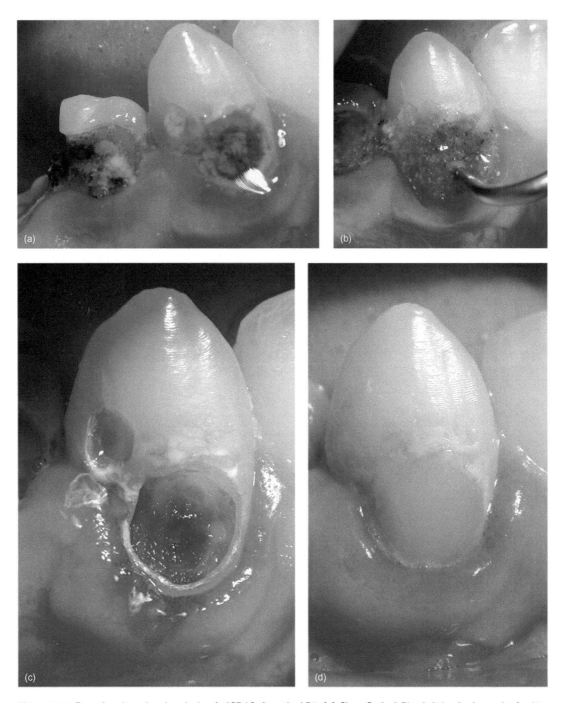

Figure 5.40 Buccal cavitated carious lesion (mICDAS 4) on the LR3. **(a)** Clear Carisolv™ gel sitting in the cavity for 30 s prior to mechanical agitation. **(b)** Gel and carious dentine agitated with a mace tip hand instrument using tooth-brushing force. Note how the caries-infected dentine 'emulsifies' into the gel, making it cloudy. A repeat application of gel was required in this case to obtain suitable carious dentine removal. No local anaesthetic or rubber dam was required. **(c)** Final cavities before restoration. There has been no direct exposure of the pulp, even though caries excavation is deep. Caries-affected dentine (scratchy but sticky/flaky) has been retained around the gingival margins in this case, along with an intact periphery of enamel (prepared using chisels/gingival margin trimmers; see Figure 5.25). (See also Section 5.9.) **(d)** Cavity has been restored provisionally with a glass ionomer cement (GIC), during the stabilization phase of the care plan (see Chapter 3).

Q5.7: Look at Figure 5.40. Why was the decision taken to retain such relatively large quantities of caries-affected dentine, especially at the gingival periphery of this particular lesion?

5.9 Minimally invasive operative management of the carious lesion

5.9.1 Rationale

The vital aspects of prevention/control of disease and patient management have been discussed in Chapters 3 and 4. There are important factors that will influence the decision to intervene operatively to treat a carious lesion:

- *Alleviate pain/'protect' the pulp*: caries removal and a sedative dressing/definitive sealed restoration can remove the symptoms of an acute, reversible pulpitis and allow the dentine–pulp complex to react and heal.

- *Restore form, function, and appearance*: a large cavitated lesion will weaken the tooth, impeding normal mastication. Smaller unsightly lesions in the anterior aesthetic zone may require operative intervention, rather than preventive measures alone, for reasons of appearance affecting the patient's inclination to smile, and ultimately their self-confidence.

- *Aid plaque control*: rough/cavitated tooth surfaces may be difficult for the high-risk patient to keep plaque-free (especially in deep occlusal pits/fissures or proximally).

- *The patient's caries risk assessment/prediction*: relatively small, early lesions in a high-risk patient with poor plaque control where repeated preventive management has been unsuccessful may require operative intervention, whereas in a lower-risk patient these same lesions may benefit from non-operative control measures (see Chapter 4). This is particularly relevant if previous preventive regimens have failed and lesions are progressing actively.

5.9.2 Minimally invasive dentistry

This is an essential part of the overall minimum intervention caries management philosophy followed in this book and dental practice—an approach where the oral healthcare team bases its individualized patient care on early detection of disease, risk assessment, diagnosis, and prevention/control of further disease with tailored recall appointment frequencies (see Chapters 3 and 9). When operative intervention is required for the reasons mentioned previously, the approach should be *minimally invasive*, that is:

1. excavation of the unrepairable, diseased enamel and dentine only, keeping cavities as small as possible and preserving sound and repairable tissue where possible

2. physically and chemically modifying/optimizing the remaining cavity walls in order to

3. restore cavities with suitable adhesive materials which will:
   - support and strengthen the remaining tooth structure
   - promote remineralization and potentially have antibacterial activity
   - seal off any remaining bacteria from their nutrient supply, thereby arresting the caries process in the residual caries retained within the cavity depths

- restore appearance, form, and function with appropriate long-term success.

In order for this minimally invasive approach to be successful, an integration of your knowledge of histology with the chemistry and handling of dental materials is essential. In addition, it is vital that the patient understands their responsibility for controlling and preventing further disease progression, as discussed in Chapter 4. Remember that 'drilling and filling' teeth does not cure caries! Any restoration placed is only ever as good as the operator placing it and the patient looking after it. In modern dental practice, it is imperative that detailed written records are kept highlighting all of this.

The decision-making process and execution of minimally invasive caries excavation/cavity preparation can be divided into the stages described in the flowchart in Figure 5.41, and will be discussed in Section 5.9.3.

5.9.3 Enamel preparation

The aims of cutting through enamel when minimally invasively operatively managing a carious lesion are to:

1. gain visual/instrumentation access to the full extent of the deeper carious dentine requiring removal

2. remove demineralized, weakened (and often unsightly frosty white) carious enamel

3. create a sound peripheral enamel margin to which an adhesive restorative material can bond and form a seal.

Figure 5.42 shows a histological cross-section through a cavitated, mICDAS 4 lesion with unsupported and demineralized enamel, and the extent of enamel preparation required. These margins may be bevelled lightly to increase the surface area for adhesion. Figure 5.43 shows the clinical occlusal appearance of such enamel removal using a diamond or TC bur in an air-turbine handpiece. This cutting process must be undertaken with only gentle pressure, avoiding the use of coarse grit diamond burs, so as not to cause excessive chipping or cracking of the remaining structure (see Figure 5.34).

Direct visual/instrumentation access to occlusal, buccal, and lingual/palatal carious surfaces is relatively straightforward with good soft tissue retraction and intra-oral lighting. Posterior proximal surface lesions (mesial and distal) can be more awkward, and approaches here would include the following:

- Occlusally, accessing initially just medial to the affected marginal ridge and eventually sacrificing it, thereby creating a proximal box (see Chapter 8).

- Occlusally, accessing medial to the marginal ridge, directing the bur towards the proximal lesion, *tunnelling* beneath the marginal ridge, and conserving it. This is only successful clinically if the lesion is sufficiently small, and it might then be debated whether operative intervention is appropriate in the first place! There is also a high risk of fracture of the weakened marginal ridge enamel in service, following restoration with a suitably flowable adhesive restorative material.

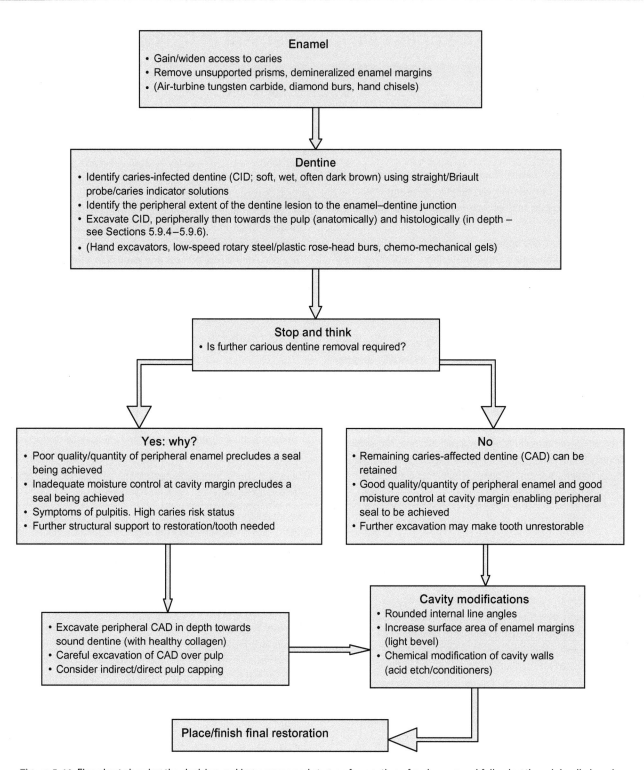

Figure 5.41 Flowchart showing the decision-making process and stages of execution of caries removal following the minimally invasive approach. These stages will be discussed in detail in Section 5.9.3.

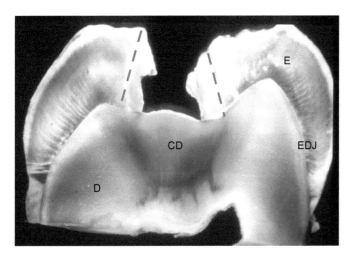

Figure 5.42 A thin mesio-distal longitudinal section through a cavitated lesion (mICDAS 4) viewed in reflected light. Note the demineralized, overhanging enamel bordering the cavity, with the undermining spread of the dentine lesion at the EDJ (see Chapter 1). The red broken lines indicate the extent of enamel removal required in order to achieve a sound enamel margin with supported prism structure, suitable for affording a seal with an adhesive restorative material while still permitting access to the underlying carious dentine. E, enamel; D, dentine; CD, carious dentine; EDJ, enamel–dentine junction.

Q5.8: Look at Figure 5.42. What is the name given to the appearance of the alternate light and dark striping evident in the inner third of enamel, arising from the EDJ and radiating towards the tooth surface?

- Buccally/lingually/palatally, especially if the tooth is rotated and has undergone some gingival recession. Tunnelling from these aspects can result in successful management as long as the lesion is not too extensive, and effective moisture and cavity margin control can be achieved.

- Directly mesial or distal, if the adjacent tooth is missing and space is present to permit direct visual/instrumentation access.

Anterior proximal lesions are approached conventionally from the lingual/palatal aspect to maintain the aesthetics of the natural labial enamel. However, minimally invasive tooth preservation principles would argue that a labial approach might be appropriate if this led to the least amount of healthy tooth tissue being destroyed. In the modern era of high-quality aesthetic direct adhesive restorative materials, this is an approach that can be encouraged, as good operator clinical skills can achieve a high-quality aesthetic result.

5.9.4 Carious dentine removal

When excavating dentine caries, careful consideration must be given to both of the following:

- 'anatomical extent' of the lesion (i.e. the lateral extent from the EDJ lesion periphery across to the caries overlying the pulp)

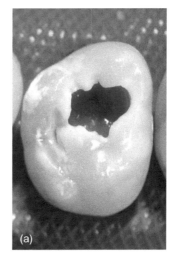
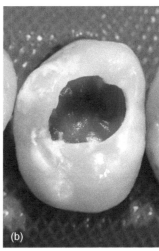

Figure 5.43 An occlusal cavitated carious lesion UR7 (mICDAS 4). **(a)** The lesion at presentation with frosty white demineralized, friable, and unsupported enamel at the cavity margin with carious dentine visible. **(b)** Enamel access has been widened by removal of the weakened peripheral enamel using a diamond bur in an air-turbine handpiece for < 5 s. The margin has been bevelled lightly.

- 'histological depth' of the lesion (i.e. the collagen and mineral content of caries-infected dentine vs. caries-affected dentine vs. sound dentine) (see Chapter 1).

Dentine caries removal must be tailored to the individual lesion, tooth, and patient. Following the minimally invasive approach, smaller cavities and restorations are created with the following benefits, ultimately leading to restorations with increased longevity and, more importantly, reduced tissue destruction and increased tooth longevity:

- Adhesive restorative materials are often easier to handle and place without voids in smaller quantities.

- Moisture control, cavity margin seal, and finish can be better regulated.

- The restored crown is often strengthened due to greater retention of natural, repairable tooth structure.

- It is simpler, and therefore results in improved patient care and maintenance.

5.9.5 Peripheral caries (EDJ)

Prevention of microleakage and subsequent recurrent caries at the cavity margin or caries progression beneath a restoration depends on the seal formed between the restoration and tooth structure at the periphery of the cavity.

- Histologically, the optimal peripheral seal achieved will be at the interface between the adhesive restorative material and sound enamel > sound dentine > caries-affected dentine > caries-infected dentine/carious enamel (the latter two being the least satisfactory and not recommended).

- The adhesive seal is created optimally between an adhesive restoration and histologically sound enamel. Therefore if sound enamel lines the entire periphery of the cavity, and moisture control is optimal (e.g.

an occlusal cavity), limited quantities of brown-discoloured, repairable, caries-affected dentine may be retained at the EDJ. However, this should be removed selectively, down to deeper sound dentine, if there is a risk that the brown discoloration may shine through the restoration, thus jeopardizing the aesthetic outcome (especially in the anterior aesthetic zone, canine–canine).

- If minimal/no enamel is present at the EDJ after peripheral caries removal, and adequate moisture control cannot be guaranteed (e.g. cervical or proximal lesion, base of a proximal box preparation close to the gingival margin), sound dentine is a prerequisite at the EDJ in an attempt to maximize the bond and adhesive seal between the peripheral dentine and final restoration. However, if this means extending the cavity a long way subgingivally, consideration must be given to the long-term success rate of the final restoration and ultimately the final restorability of the tooth in question (see Figure 5.40).

- Distinguishing between caries-infected, caries-affected, and sound dentine is a rather subjective skill, and the operator usually uses differential tactile judgement (see Table 5.7). Brown discoloration of the dentine at the EDJ is an indicator neither of its infectivity nor of the need for its removal (unless in the anterior aesthetic zone).

- In no clinical situation should caries-infected dentine be retained at the EDJ, as this dentine is essentially necrotic and cannot be adhered to or a seal achieved. It is also too soft to physically support a rigid restoration under occlusal load.

- Instruments commonly used include hand excavators or steel rose-head burs in a low-speed handpiece. Other technologies might include chemo-mechanical agents (see Table 5.5).

5.9.6 Caries overlying the pulp

When excavating dentine caries overlying the pulp, consideration must be given to its *proximity* to the pulp (see Section 5.11) and any *symptoms*.

- Where a peripheral seal can be achieved (enamel margins intact) and pulp symptoms are not present, quantities of caries-affected dentine may be retained overlying the pulp, thereby reducing the risk of pulp exposure. Clinical evidence now shows that affected dentine provides better indirect pulp protection than any artificial restorative material in this situation.

- If the dentine lesion has only penetrated into the middle third of dentine radiographically, thanks to tertiary dentine being laid down at the dentine–pulp border, excavation to sound dentine may be achievable to improve the adhesive bond and seal (especially if the enamel margins are not intact).

- Where chronic pulp symptoms persist along with radiographic changes at the apex, caries excavation needs to be complete, exposing the pulp chamber and its necrotic contents if necessary with a view to the continuation of endodontic treatment.

Table 5.6 summarizes the interlinked factors that affect the decision to remove/retain carious dentine. It must be understood that there is no absolute correct or incorrect amount of caries that should be excavated, but whatever decision is made by the operator, it should be made for *pragmatic*, *justifiable*, and *documented* reasons. Different quantities of caries can be removed or retained in different parts of the same

---

Table 5.6 A summary of the interrelating factors that affect the decision about how much dentine caries to excavate (infected vs. affected vs. sound)

Factors affecting amount of carious dentine removed	Comments 'GIC, glass ionomer cement'
Patient's caries risk	High-risk, uncontrolled caries progression, unsuccessful prevention regimes: lesions may be treated with excavation to sound dentine where possible. Important for operator and patient to appreciate the reduced longevity of the tooth–restoration complex due to the lack of patient adherence to preventive strategies (see Chapter 9)
Patient/oral factors	Limited oral opening, physical/mental disabilities can affect visual/instrument access directly/indirectly. Broken down/rotated/partially erupted teeth can hinder rubber dam placement. Sedation/general anaesthesia may be required
Pulp vitality (sensibility)	Chronic symptoms of an irreversible pulpitis will mean pulp extirpation after complete caries removal to sound dentine
Pulp proximity	If no/limited acute pulp symptoms, CAD retained over the pulpal aspect of cavity to allow remineralization from dentine–pulp complex—*indirect pulp capping/protection*
Remaining coronal tooth structure	Sufficient supragingival tooth structure must remain to support the restoration long term. Excavation to sound dentine should not compromise the physical/adhesive properties of the restorative material (e.g. deep peripheral excavation to sound dentine resulting in a cavity margin of > 2 mm subgingivally, compromising moisture control and marginal adaptation)
Material factors	Retention mechanisms—mechanical, micro-mechanical, chemical adhesion. An adverse oral environment can affect the set and physical properties of some materials (e.g. GICs in xerostomia)

CAD, caries-affected dentine.

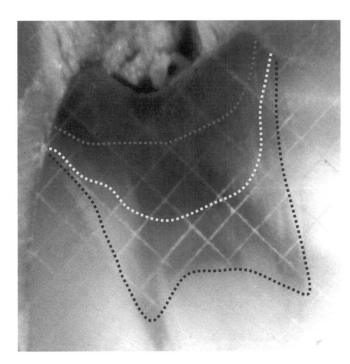

Figure 5.44 A cavitated dentine lesion (mICDAS 3/4) showing the colour gradation from the superficial caries-infected dentine subjacent to the EDJ through to the deeper levels of caries-affected dentine, including the translucent zone and sound dentine. Three positions have been indicated for potential caries excavation endpoints: white line—excavation to sound dentine at EDJ and pulpal aspect; green line—less invasive excavation retaining stained dentine at the EDJ and affected dentine over the pulp; blue line—minimally invasive excavation finishing on sound enamel at the EDJ and infected/affected dentine over the pulp. Note how all of the potential endpoints finish on sound enamel, so providing a sealed margin. None of these endpoints are right or wrong, but it is essential that the histology at each level is appreciated in order to enable a successful adhesive restoration to be placed.

> **Q5.9:** Which of the three levels do you think would be best to stop caries removal in the lesion shown in Figure 5.44?

cavity. Figure 5.44 highlights this variation in dentine caries removal, showing three levels of potential excavation endpoint, depending on the combined outcome of the factors discussed in Table 5.6.

5.9.7 Distinguishing the zones of carious dentine

The clinical discrimination between caries-infected, caries-affected, and sound dentine is at present a subjective skill gained by using a combination of an understanding of caries histology and clinical experience. These boundaries are not clearly defined; the histological and bacterial changes occur throughout the whole lesion as a continuum from superficial to deeper layers, with different rates of progression within the individual lesion itself. Table 5.7 summarizes the techniques available—both clinical and through research development—to help to enable the operator to distinguish these important 'histological' layers.

From the table it can be seen that none are truly objective, with interpretation required to decide the excavation endpoint and linked to the factors discussed in Table 5.6.

5.9.8 'Stepwise excavation' and the atraumatic restorative technique (ART)

These two operative techniques are the original and more modern application, respectively, of the minimally invasive biological approach to managing larger cavitated carious lesions. Both can use simple hand instrumentation (spoon-shaped excavators) to remove the necrotic, superficial layer of caries-infected dentine and some caries-affected dentine also if required (see Figure 5.45). The two stages of the original stepwise excavation procedure included the placement of a calcium hydroxide lining and a temporary zinc polycarboxylate cement restoration. Between 6 and 9 months later, this restoration was removed completely, exposing the remaining, now arrested caries-affected dentine (darker, harder, and dryer) and newly deposited tertiary dentine at the pulp–dentine border. The residual stained dentine was now removed

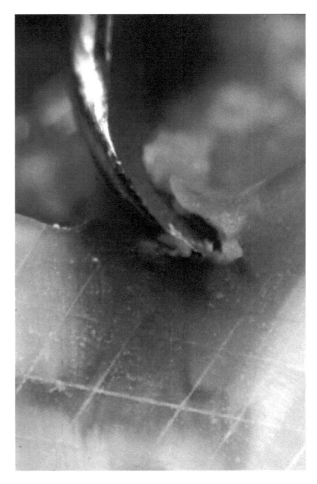

Figure 5.45 Hand excavator scooping through necrotic, soft caries-infected dentine once the enamel access has been widened (reference grid lines on the dentine face were placed for experimental purposes).

Table 5.7 Clinical and research methods used to help to discriminate clinically between the three histological zones of carious dentine (infected, affected, and sound). Note that these zones do not have distinct boundaries, but have a gradient of histological/bacterial change through them from the enamel–dentine junction (EDJ) to the pulp (see Chapter 1)

Discriminating methods		Caries-infected dentine	Caries-affected dentine	Sound dentine
Clinical	Visual	Often a colour gradient from (see Figure 5.44): Dark brown → paler brown/translucent → yellow/white Difficult to judge clinically/OK when examining a sectioned lesion (research)		
	Tactile	Soft/sticky feel with a sharp dental probe (straight or Briault)	Both sticky/flaky and scratchy feel	Scratchy feel to a sharp dental probe
	Caries detector dyes	'Fusayama' dyes—based on propylene-glycol, collagen-based stain. Attempts to discriminate infected vs. affected, but research has shown that these dyes stain deeper collagen and permeate into affected/sound dentine zones, often leading to cavity over-preparation		
Research	Bacterial dyes	Dyes under research development reacting to bacterial redox by-products, using their concentration gradient drop from infected through affected to sound dentine. Have potential to be zone-selective		
	Fluorescence	Research into the natural fluorescence of dentine caries using confocal fibre-optic microendoscopy/fluorescence lifetime imaging (FLIM) indicates a discriminating level of fluorescence of infected dentine. A technique that might be developed for *in-vivo* use in the future		

using a steel rose-head bur in a low-speed handpiece, and a final amalgam restoration was placed.

The more recently described single-step ART proposes restoring the cavity with chemically adhesive, high-viscosity glass ionomer cement (GIC), forming a better adaptive seal to the remaining tooth structure (see Chapter 7) after the use of simple hand excavators to gain access to and remove the caries-infected dentine. Subsequently, this provisional restoration does not require complete replacement as in the original stepwise excavation procedure, as the arrested caries-affected dentine is sealed off from its nutrient supply. However, occlusal resurfacing of the GIC may be necessary after 2 to 3 years due to its wear and partial dissolution. This can be accomplished by cutting back the exposed worn GIC surface by up to 2 mm in depth, and bonding a layer of resin composite on to the freshly exposed, mature GIC—an *adhesive layered, laminate* or *'sandwich' restoration*

(see Chapters 7 and 8). Indeed, systematic reviews of partial/incomplete minimally invasive caries removal have highlighted how the one-stage procedure with no re-entry stage, that seals in residual affected dentine, results in significantly less pulp exposures than the original two-step stepwise excavation procedure. This finding was the result of an increase in pulp exposures in the second re-entry procedure where deeper dentine was removed (forcibly and unnecessarily) too close to the pulp.

Both stepwise excavation and ART follow the underpinning principles of minimally invasive dentistry. As this is a more accepted contemporary rationale for operative caries management, these terminologies are now becoming redundant as current adhesive dental materials are more capable of sealing in and potentially rehabilitating diseased tissue.

5.10 Cavity modification

Once caries removal has been achieved, the dentist needs to stop, think, and decide which restorative material to use, and then modify the remaining cavity accordingly, if required (see Figure 5.46). These changes may be necessary to improve the retentive properties or to maximize the material properties (e.g. bulk/margin strength or fracture resistance).

- *Retention*: the property of a cavity that resists displacement of the restoration in the direction of its insertion.

- *Cavity support*: the cavity property that prevents displacement (or fracture) of the restoration in any other direction, including internal dislodgement within the cavity itself. This feature relates to the morphology of cavity walls/floors and rounded internal line angles.

Table 5.8 outlines the different macro- (bur-induced) or micro-modifications (chemically induced) dependent on the restorative material to be used.

Table 5.8 Potential cavity modifications required after caries removal, depending on the material chosen to restore the cavity*

Restorative material	Cavity modification		Comments
Resin composite/GIC	macro	Enamel margin bevel (short/long)	Removes grossly unsupported prisms Increases surface area for bond/seal Provides a sound enamel surface to facilitate optimal adhesive bonding (see Figures 5.42, 5.43, and 5.46b)
All	macro	Rounded internal line angles	Reduces both internal stresses and risk of crack propagation within the restoration (see Figures 5.46, 5.47, 5.48, 5.49, 5.50)
Resin composite	micro	Enamel acid etch	37% orthophosphoric acid removes smear layer, and selectively demineralizes prisms, creating micro-mechanical undercuts for resin retention
GIC	micro	Dentine conditioner	10% polyacrylic/citric acids modify or remove smear layer, preparing the surface for chemical adhesion (Ca^{2+})
Amalgam	macro	Cavity undercuts, grooves, slots, flat surfaces	Cavities with wider bases than orifices are required for retention of amalgam—undercuts. Slots/grooves help to prevent further displacement of the restoration (see Figures 5.48 and 5.49) Flat cavity surfaces with rounded internal line angles help to improve the internal cavity support (see Figure 5.50)
All	macro	Pulp chamber	In endodontically treated teeth, the pulp chamber is used to add bulk and retentive features/increased surface area for the coronal restoration
Amalgam	macro	Nayyar core	Packing the coronally flared 2–3 mm of endodontically treated root canals to improve core retention
Gold, porcelain, resin composite (indirect restorations)	macro	Long marginal taper	Divergent tapered margins (7–10°) used to improve retentive features of indirect restorations (see Chapter 6)

*The modifications have been classified as macro (those created using a bur) or micro (those created using chemicals). See Chapter 7 for a description of the material science and Chapter 8 for practical considerations.

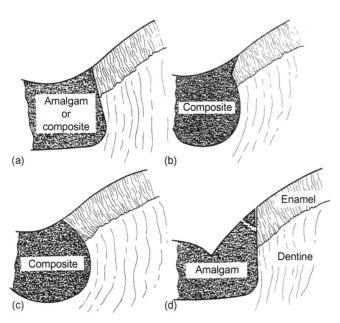

(a)

(b)

(c)

(d)

Enamel

Dentine

Amalgam or composite

Composite

Composite

Amalgam

Figure 5.46 Diagrams outlining the different restoration margin angles and cavo-surface angles that are suited to different restorative materials. **(a)** Amalgam and resin composite margins require bulk for strength, so 90° restoration margin angles and cavo-surface angles will ensure sufficient intrinsic strength of both the restoration margin and cavity edge. **(b)** Resin composites adhere and support enamel to a degree, so light bevelling of the enamel surface can increase the surface area for adhesive bonding while also removing any potentially unsupported enamel prisms at the cavity edge **(c)**. **(d)** If the amalgam margin angle is too acute, the amalgam margin may be weakened sufficiently for marginal fracture to occur under occlusal loading. Note the internal rounded line angles in all of the cavities depicted.

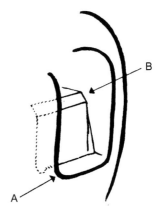

B

A

Figure 5.47 Diagram indicating the internal bevelling/rounding off of the internal line angles between adjacent internal cavity surfaces (A and B). This reduces the risk of crack propagation within the restorative material.

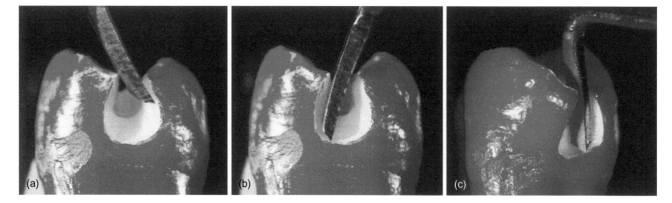

(a)

(b)

(c)

Figure 5.48 (a–c) Proximal box cavity prepared with undercuts (a wider base and a narrower occlusal opening) to prevent displacement of the restoration (amalgam) occlusally from its path of insertion.

Q5.10: Which hand instrument is shown in Figure 5.48?

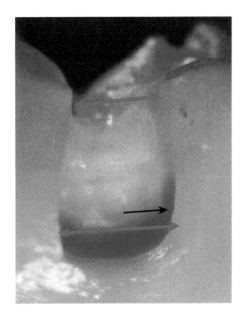

Figure 5.49 A proximal box cavity prepared with occlusal undercuts (a wider base and a narrow occlusal opening—thick red arrows) to prevent displacement of the restoration (amalgam) from its path of insertion occlusally. Note the rounded internal line angles. The thin black arrow shows the placement of a groove at the junction between the buccal wall of the box and the pulpal wall, so providing stability (resistance) to proximal displacement.

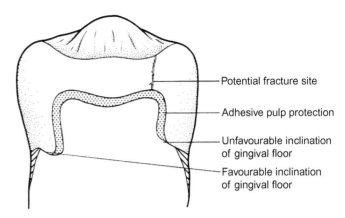

Figure 5.50 Potential problems of the morphology of cavity walls and floor, requiring modification. Rounded internal line angles reduce the risk of crack propagation and eventual restoration fracture of rigid materials (e.g. amalgam). Use of a rose-head bur to remove carious dentine tends to create the cavity floor morphology on the left, but care must be taken to remove any very prominent unsupported enamel lip at the periphery. The floor morphology on the right offers limited support to the final restoration and should be avoided.

5.11 Pulp protection

5.11.1 Rationale

The final and most important consideration along with any cavity modifications, prior to placing the restoration, is the long-term pulp status. This is linked to pulp *signs and symptoms* and *cavity proximity* to the pulp. Assuming that the symptoms and signs of pulp sensibility indicate a histologically viable pulp (see Chapter 3), the pulp tissues may require protection from:

- bacteria/toxins
- chemicals leaching from the restorative materials (e.g. unconverted resin monomers from resin composite restoratives, acid etchant)
- thermal and/or electrical stimulation via conductance through the overlying restoration.

If the floor of the cavity is close to the pulp but the pulp chamber has not been breached during minimally invasive caries removal, this protection can be afforded by a process termed *indirect pulp capping (IPC)*. If a small breach, or *pulp exposure*, has occurred (usually no wider than the tip of a Williams periodontal probe), created either iatrogenically or by the caries process, a *direct pulp cap (DPC)* may be placed in an attempt to maintain pulp viability, but the patient must be warned that this is not guaranteed, especially when this is a consequence of a deep carious lesion (see Figure 5.51).

5.11.2 Terminology

There are two older terms used in the dental literature to describe this form of material-based pulp protection where an exposure has not occurred—*cavity lining* and *structural base*. These terms were coined when amalgam was the only material of choice to restore cavities long term and it was thought that the pulp required an 'insulating' layer between it and the metal-based restoration. The excessively large, undercut cavities designed for amalgam could be reduced in size artificially by placing zinc oxide-based plastic materials as 'structural bases', on to which was packed a reduced volume of amalgam. In the contemporary era of minimally invasive operative dentistry, these terms should no longer be used, so as to avoid confusion.

5.11.3 Materials

Materials used for both IPC and DPC should ideally:

- be bactericidal (able to kill bacteria)/bacteriostatic (able to prevent them from multiplying)
- be mildly irritant to the pulp, to stimulate tertiary dentine bridge formation (usually via pH changes)
- be adhesive in order to effect a bond and seal
- not dissolve away over time
- be easily applied and strong in thin section

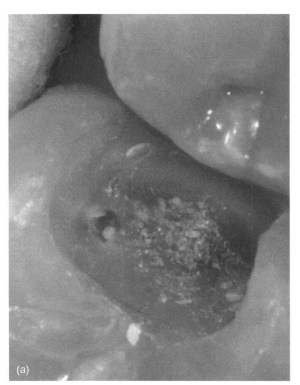
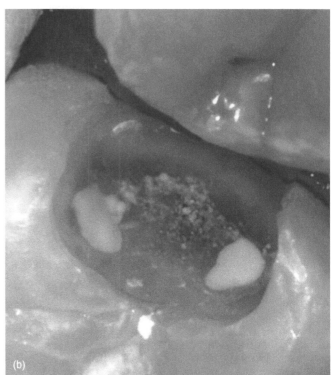

Figure 5.51 **(a)** Caries excavated from a proximal lesion in a vital tooth with residual caries-affected dentine evident on the pulpal aspect of the cavity. Note the spot of blood exuding from a small carious exposure through the pulp horn. **(b)** Setting calcium hydroxide has been placed over the small pulp exposures. (Courtesy of L. Mackenzie.)

Q5.11: After placing the direct pulp cap as shown in Figure 5.51, what are the next steps in the restoration of this cavity?

- be able to infiltrate ionically into the remaining dentine overlying the pulp, thereby strengthening/reinforcing it
- be biocompatible with the pulp and the overlying restorative material.

Clinical dental materials used for IPC and DPC (see Chapter 7) include:

- glass ionomer cements
- dentine bonding agents
- setting calcium hydroxide
- tricalcium silicate cements (mineralized trioxide aggregate (MTA), Biodentine™).

The first two materials in the previous list fulfil the majority of the criteria for an ideal IPC mentioned earlier. When using these adhesive materials as the final restorative solution, it can be argued that a separate thin layer of pulp protection is not necessary, as the properties are 'built in' to the bulk restorative material itself. Setting calcium hydroxide cements have been used for many years as pulp protection beneath amalgam restorations, but in recent times much more sparingly. The authors cannot suggest any positive indications for their use beneath adhesive restorations as an IPC. GICs and resin-based cements

are being used increasingly in bonded amalgam restorations, so again the use of calcium hydroxide is ever more limited in this regard. As a DPC, the alkaline pH of calcium hydroxide still has a use as an inflammatory stimulant for pulp odontoblasts to produce tertiary dentine and so close the exposure. Unset MTA is primarily calcium oxide in the form of tricalcium silicate, dicalcium silicate, and tricalcium aluminate, with bismuth oxide added for radio-opacity. Several studies indicate its potential use as a DPC, as it increases the concentration of available calcium hydroxide, the primary reaction product between MTA and water, and provides a seal. However, its high solubility, long setting time (up to 3 hours), and expense are disadvantages. Both setting calcium hydroxide cements and MTA need a second protective covering prior to placing the final restoration. This is conventionally a GIC/resin-modified (RM)-GIC material (see Chapter 7). A faster-setting calcium tri-silicate restorative cement, Biodentine™, now exists, that incorporates the pulp protection properties within its bulk restoration (see Chapter 7).

Interestingly, clinical evidence now shows that retained caries-affected dentine overlying acutely inflamed pulps provides the optimum qualities of indirect pulp protection as long as the overlying adhesive restoration affords an adequate seal and the patient can maintain adequate oral hygiene and other preventive measures.

5.12 Dental matrices

(See also Chapter 8.) Cavities created with missing proximal walls present a technical problem when it comes to placing a direct plastic restorative material, as there is nothing to contain the restoration within the cavity or to prevent poor marginal adaptation (ledges, overhangs). *Circumferential* matrix bands, with retainers (e.g. reusable Siqveland and Tofflemire, disposable AutoMatrix and Omni-matrix; see Figure 5.52a) or without (e.g. copper rings, AutoMatrix or SuperMat matrices; see Figure 5.52b), or *sectional* matrix bands have been developed to rectify this problem (Palodent, Composi-Tight, V-Ring, QuickMat, among others). Traditional dental matrix systems consist of two components:

- *Single-use matrix band*: thin metal or clear plastic band of varying widths and gauges (30–50 μm) used to form the missing wall of the cavity. More rigid and wider bands used posteriorly (metal), and narrower, pliable, transparent plastic bands used anteriorly (for resin composites).

- *Retainer*: a device used to tighten and hold circumferential matrix bands in place proximally. These can be sterilized and used again. Sectional matrix systems have oval/round ring retainers with curved tines to adapt the matrix to the proximal tooth contour (see Figure 5.53).

5.12.1 Clinical tips

- Cervical margin adaptation of the band to the tooth is essential to prevent ledges or overhangs of excess restorative material, often requiring the use of wooden/plastic wedges in the interproximal space.

- Tight interdental contact points may need to be opened slightly by causing differential movement of the adjacent teeth within their periodontal ligament spaces. This is accomplished by pre-wedging using wooden wedges for a few minutes prior to placing the band.

- Sectional matrices may be of benefit in situations where teeth are rotated or tilted, thus making the placement of circumferential bands more difficult.

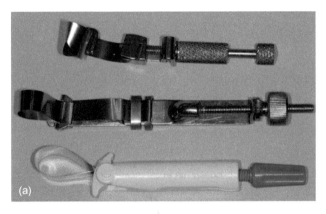 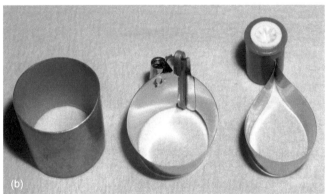

Figure 5.52 **(a)** Three examples of circumferential metal matrix bands with retainers. Top: Tofflemire retainer with precurved matrix band; middle: Siqveland retainer with matrix band; bottom: Omni-matrix disposable system. **(b)** Three examples of circumferential matrix bands without retainers: copper ring, AutoMatrix®, and SuperMat® systems.

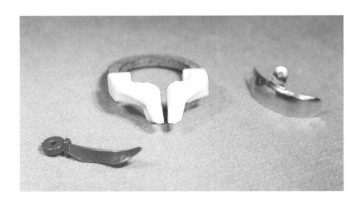

Figure 5.53 A precurved and contoured single-use sectional metal matrix band (right) with a plastic gingivally contoured wedge (left) and the oval ring retainer with curved tines (middle) to adapt the band to the approximal surface of the tooth. The retainer can be sterilized.

- Sectional bands are more adaptable to gain well-contoured proximal surfaces and contact areas.

- Circumferential bands can be more painful for the patient to endure than equivalent sectional bands.

- Clear plastic bands/wedges can be used when placing resin composite restorations to permit light penetration to the depths of the proximal cavity when curing the material.

- Rubber dam clamps may have to be removed prior to placing matrix bands.

- Anteriorly, if contact areas are tight and the flexible, clear plastic matrix band refuses to pass through incisally, the corner of the band can be cut to a point and passed cervically beneath the contact and then lifted incisally through it.

5.13 Temporary (intermediate) restorations

5.13.1 Definitions

A *temporary restoration* is one that is placed for short-term use (usually days or weeks), often between appointments in a course of ongoing definitive treatment (e.g. caries stabilization, multi-visit root canal treatment, simple fixed prosthodontics).

A *provisional restoration* is one that is placed for short/medium-term duration (weeks or months) where diagnostic value is gained from placing the restoration (e.g. complex fixed prosthodontic treatment when reorganizing a patient's occlusion or adjusting the vertical dimension of the patient's occlusion (see later); stabilizing caries to negate symptoms).

The dental material science of temporary restorations (GIC, zinc oxide eugenol, and zinc polycarboxylates) is covered in Chapter 7. Eugenol-containing temporary restorations should be avoided in cavities where the final restoration to be placed is a resin composite, as the eugenol adversely affects the resin's polymerization chemistry.

5.13.2 Clinical tips

- Care must be taken when placing temporary restorations to replicate the occlusion and marginal adaptation of the restoration.
- Zinc oxide-based materials have a relatively poor appearance, so in the anterior aesthetic zone the use of GIC-based materials might be considered.
- Patients must be made fully aware of the reason for and function of the temporary restoration.
- Adequate time must be allocated in the clinical appointment to place temporary restorations. Poor-quality marginal adaptation of temporaries can lead to further marginal staining, plaque accumulation, and gingival inflammation/bleeding which in turn often worsens the patient's oral hygiene procedures.
- Frustratingly, if temporary/provisional restorations have optimal aesthetics, the patient may not wish to have them replaced with their definitive counterparts!

5.14 Principles of dental occlusion

In order to successfully restore dental function in the long term, an understanding of human dental occlusion is of primary importance. This subject is complex, and many textbooks exist that discuss these complexities and their clinical relevance. The occlusal contacts between the maxillary and mandibular dentition are affected by the skeletal base relationship (condylar head vs. slope of the articular eminence, glenoid fossa), development of the maxilla and mandible, and direct factors influencing the development, position, and shape of the teeth themselves. Analysis of occlusion is critical in both the *conformative* and *reorganizational* approaches to managing dental care.

5.14.1 Definitions

Conformative approach

This approach to planning and placing restorations ensures that the pre-existing occlusal relationships are not altered in any of the three planes (antero-posterior, vertical, and horizontal). It is essential therefore to analyse aspects of the occlusion prior to commencing, so that the final restorations fit into the existing scheme. This approach most often applies when placing single or multiple plastic, direct restorations.

Reorganizational approach

This approach involves changes in occlusion, and is often undertaken when rehabilitating major occlusal discrepancies caused by tilting or over-eruption of teeth resulting in premature occlusal interference contacts and/or distortion of the occlusal planes causing reduced space into which to place definitive restorations. Here again considerable planning with the use of provisional restorations is required in order to calculate the tolerances of changing the occlusion. This approach is usually indicated in complex cases often involving the use of indirect restorations (crowns, bridges, dentures, or implants), and is beyond the scope of this particular textbook.

5.14.2 Terminology

The commonly used terminology and recorded positions of occlusal analysis are described in Table 5.9. QR code image 5.2 will take you to a glossary of prosthodontic terms.

 QR code image 5.2. Scan this code with your mobile device to access a glossary of prosthodontic terms.

www.thejpd.org/article/S0022-39(13)0500175-7/fulltext

5.14.3 Occlusal registration techniques

The various static and dynamic relationships of the patient's occlusion should be analysed before starting any restorative procedure in the conformative approach to dental care provision, as well as checking again after the restoration(s) has been completed. There are many different clinical techniques available for checking direct occlusal contact relationships in the patient's mouth:

- *Articulating paper*: thickness in the range 40–200 μm; different colours that show up contact areas between cusp inclines and fossae on occlusion (see Figure 5.54).

Table 5.9 Various occlusal relationships, their definitions, and their relevance to restorative dentistry

Occlusal relationship	Definition	Diagram/comments
Intercuspal position (ICP) (static)	The occlusal relationship where there is maximum cusp interdigitation between the maxillary and mandibular teeth	Not always clinically reproducible, and can be affected by occlusal interferences
Occlusal vertical dimension (OVD) (static)	The vertical relationship between the maxilla and mandible with the teeth in ICP	Can be reduced by tooth wear, missing teeth Can be compensated biologically by over-eruption of teeth/dento-alveolar compensation
Rest position (RP) (static)	The vertical relationship between the maxilla and mandible when resting comfortably in an upright position with relaxed facial musculature	Achieved after swallowing/yawning. Teeth usually slightly apart
Freeway space (FS) (static)	The vertical dimension difference between RP and OVD (ranges 2–4 mm)	Adaptive in the dentate patient Essential consideration for the restoration of the edentate individual with complete dentures
Overjet (OJ) (static)	The horizontal distance between the maxillary and mandibular incisal edges in ICP	
Overbite (OB) (static)	The vertical distance between the maxillary and mandibular incisal edges in ICP No vertical overlap can lead to an edge–edge incisal relationship or an anterior open bite (AOB)	
Retruded contact position (RCP) (dynamic)	The most retruded position of the mandible when there is initial cusp contact (described as the relationship where the condylar heads are rearmost within their glenoid fossae and rotate about their terminal hinge axis or *centric relation*)	A clinically reproducible and registerable position used in the dental rehabilitation of the edentulous patient as well as in the reorganized approach in the dentate patient
Lateral excursions (dynamic)	Occlusal relationship between the teeth when the mandible is shifted horizontally to the right or left Working side: the side to which the mandible has moved Non-working side: the side away from which the mandible has moved	Horizontal movement guided by working side: 1. palatal/labial surfaces of canines/incisors 2. cuspal inclines of premolars/molars 3. a combination of both. Horizontal movement may also be guided by non-working side contacts and condylar head–glenoid fossae relationships
Protrusion (dynamic)	The anterior/forward movement of the mandible with teeth in occlusion	Usually guided by the palatal contour of the maxillary incisors Leads to a posterior open bite—Christensen's phenomenon

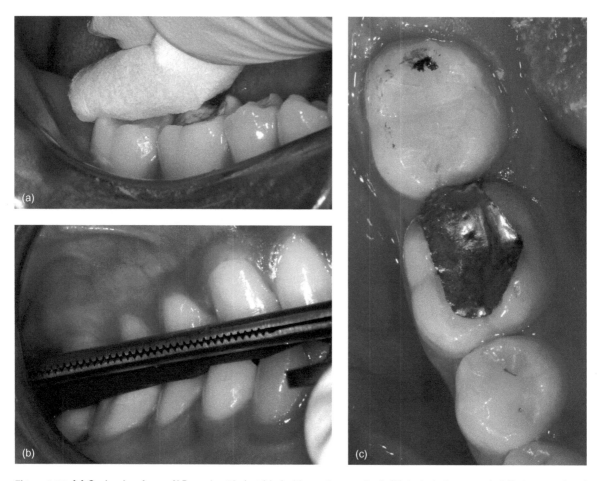

Figure 5.54 (a) Occlusal surfaces of LR quadrant being dried with a cotton wool roll. **(b)** Articulating paper held in forceps placed on occlusal surfaces and patient asked to bite together in the intercuspal position (ICP) and slide teeth left and right. **(c)** Heavy occlusal cusp–fossa contact shown on distal occlusal aspect of LR7 (red mark—ICP, black mark—lateral excursions). This can now be selectively removed with a rotary instrument.

Q5.12:

i   Why is it important to dry the teeth prior to using dental articulating paper?

ii What mandibular movements should the patient shown in Figure 5.54 be encouraged to make when checking the occlusion using articulating paper?

- *Shimstock*: articulating foil (8 μm) for the fine occlusal adjustment of coronal restorations.

- *Clinical observation*: assess dental contacts around the arch prior to removing an old/damaged restoration, and ensure that these are replicated with the new restoration, especially in the partially dentate.

5.14.4 Clinical tips

- Occlusion must be checked both *before* and *after* placement of any restoration affecting the occlusal or guidance surfaces of teeth. Different coloured articulating paper can be used in this regard. This is essential in the conformative approach to dental care provision.

- Occlusal surfaces should be dried with cotton wool rolls (see Figure 5.54a).

- Occlusion must be checked dynamically as well as statically. The patient must be asked to 'grind' their teeth side to side and back to front in order to check that the guidance paths are free from interferences.

- Even though some authorities classify the buccal cusps of the mandibular teeth and palatal cusps of the maxillary dentition as *functional cusps*, it must be realized that all cusps, ridges, and fossae have an important role to play in a harmonious dynamic occlusion.

5.15 Suggested further reading and PubMed keywords

Department of Health (2009) *Delivering Better Oral Health. An evidence- based toolkit for prevention - second edition.* London: Department of Health/BASCD.
<www.dh.gov.uk/en/Publicationsandstatistics/Publications/PublicationsPolicyAndGuidance/DH_102331>

<www.ncbi.nlm.nih.gov/pubmed/advanced>

QR code image 5.3 Try searching the following keywords on PubMed for relevant further reading. You can access PubMed by scanning the QR code image or at the address www.ncbi.nlm.nih.gov/pubmed/advanced

Keywords

BDA infection control (UK); dental infection control; Department of Health (UK); HTM01-05; minimal intervention dentistry; minimally invasive dentistry; MI Compendium; glossary of prosthodontic terms.

5.16 Answers to self-test questions

Q5.1: Can you spot the gold crown in Figure 5.7?

A: It is present on the upper right-hand side of the radiograph—the discrete radio-opacity.

Q5.2: Can you spot an important clinical omission in Figure 5.17?

A: The safety floss around the connector arm and through the holes of the clamp is missing. This aids in retrieving pieces in cases of clamp separation.

Q5.3: In which clinical situations might you use each of the probes shown in Figure 5.21?

A: Straight probe—clinical examination of restoration margins and exposed carious dentine. Briault probe—proximal surfaces, internal cavity walls. Williams probe—periodontal pocket assessment, clinical examination of tooth surfaces. Naber's probe—periodontal furcation measurement. CPITN probe—periodontal assessment, clinical examination of tooth surfaces.

Q5.4: What are the advantages of having angulations between the working head and shank of the instruments pictured in Figure 5.24?

A: To enable the operator to access all aspects of a cavity, undercut, or undermined areas as well as offsetting the handle to allow better direct visual access to instrumentation.

Q5.5: What might be the advantages and disadvantages of single-use, disposable burs?

A: Advantages—improved infection control, no maintenance required. Disadvantages—potential long-term cost, possible concerns about quality control over the precision in manufacture, availability of all types of bur.

Q5.6: What clinical situations may benefit from using air-abrasion tooth preparation?

A: Minimally invasive dentistry procedures—diagnosing and treating carious fissures in high-risk patients with unmodifiable risk factors, tooth preparation for direct labial composite veneers, all tooth surface pre-treatment prior to adhesive bonding, stain removal/refreshing surfaces of old composites, potential selective enamel/dentine caries removal (with bioactive glass particles—in development).

Q5.7: Look at Figure 5.40. Why was the decision taken to retain such relatively large quantities of caries-affected dentine, especially at the gingival periphery of this particular lesion?

A: This was a conscious decision as an intact enamel periphery was present to create an adhesive seal. If the carious dentine was removed at the EDJ (as normal) this would result in a cavity margin that would be located on root dentine at least 3–4 mm subgingivally, with no enamel present. Moisture control would then be impossible, no seal would be achievable, and the tooth/cavity would be unrestorable. By retaining this affected dentine, the tooth (dentine–pulp complex) has been given the opportunity to heal itself, with suitable input from the patient with regard to oral hygiene and dietary concerns.

Q5.8: Look at Figure 5.42. What is the name given to the appearance of the alternate light and dark striping evident in the inner third of enamel, arising from the EDJ and radiating towards the tooth surface?

A: Hunter–Schreger bands.

Q5.9: Which of the three levels do you think would be best to stop caries removal in the lesion shown in Figure 5.44?

A: Probably the second level (the green line) on caries-affected dentine where the collagen has partial structure to enable some form of dentine bonding to take place and the periphery histological status will allow a seal to be achieved, while not encroaching on the pulp and risking exposure.

Q5.10: Which hand instrument is shown in Figure 5.48?

A: Gingival margin trimmer.

Q5.11: After placing the direct pulp cap as shown in Figure 5.51, what are the next steps in the restoration of this cavity?

A: The setting calcium hydroxide should be protected with a layer of GIC/RMGIC. Then the adhesive restorative procedure can be performed—etch, bond, and placement of a resin composite restoration.

Q5.12:

i Why is it important to dry the teeth prior to using dental articulating paper?

A: To allow the ink from the paper to adhere to and mark the teeth in discrete areas of tooth–tooth contact.

ii What mandibular movements should the patient shown in Figure 5.54 be encouraged to make when checking the occlusion using articulating paper?

A: Vertical intercuspal position (the patient should be asked to bite up and down) and also lateral excursions (the patient should be asked to grind their teeth side to side to assess the cuspal inclines guiding the occlusion in these directions).

6

Principles of management of the badly broken down tooth

6.1 Causes of broken down teeth

This textbook has covered the common causes of broken down teeth: dental caries, tooth wear, and trauma. In addition, long-term failure of parts, or all, of the existing tooth–restoration complex can be significant and may require further operative intervention for its successful management (see Chapter 9). Many intra-coronal defects can be repaired with direct adhesive restorations, as discussed in Chapters 5 and 9. However, the situation can be complicated by the loss of significant portions of existing restoration or tooth structure (e.g. cusps, buccal/lingual walls), which influence the restorative procedures used in an attempt to maintain the tooth longevity, as well as pulp viability, for as long as possible. For direct restorations to succeed clinically, they require healthy dental tissues to aid support, retention,

and ideally provide an element of protection from excessive occlusal loads. With diminishing amounts of tooth structure to work with, greater thought and care are required to manage and prepare the remaining viable hard tissues to support and retain the larger restoration.

The *core restoration* describes the often large direct plastic restoration used to build up the clinically broken down crown. It is retained and supported by remaining tooth structure wherever possible (sometimes including the pulp chamber and posts in root canals of endodontically treated teeth). These large restorations often benefit from further overlying protection to secure their clinical longevity, by means of *indirect onlays*, and *partial or full coverage crowns*.

6.2 Clinical assessment of broken down teeth

Before carrying out a detailed clinical examination of the individual tooth and the related oral cavity, it is always important to *justify* your clinical decisions, for both operative and non-operative preventive interventions.

6.2.1 Why restore the broken down (or any) tooth?

The five key reasons for minimally invasive (MI) operative intervention are:

- to repair hard tissue damage/cavitation caused by the active, progressing caries/tooth-wear process (where non-operative prevention has failed repeatedly)
- to remove plaque stagnation areas within cavities/defects which will increase the risk of caries activity due to the lack of effective plaque removal by the patient
- to help to manage acute pulpitic pain caused by active caries by removing the bacterial biomass and sealing the defect, thereby protecting the pulp
- to restore the tooth to maintain structure and function in the dental arch
- aesthetics.

6.2.2 Is the broken down tooth restorable?

This is a very important question to answer pragmatically for the patient sitting in the dental chair at the time of consultation. It is important to manage patient expectations in this regard, as often the operative treatment required is complex technically, takes time over multiple appointments, and may be expensive. Critical issues will include the longevity and functionality of the final restoration; the patient has to appreciate the cost weighed against the clinical benefit of the treatment proposed, along with any significant risks of short-, medium-, or long-term failure. The factors that must be considered when deciding whether to restore a broken down tooth are outlined in Table 6.1. These principles must, of course, be applied to any teeth that are being restored, but are highlighted again in this chapter.

The clinical oral and dental assessment follows the guidance outlined and discussed in Chapters 2 and 3. After obtaining a comprehensive patient history and performing a clinical examination of the whole mouth, the following tooth-related factors should be determined:

- periapical radiographs to help to ascertain the periapical status, presence/absence/quality of root canal treatment (RCT), extent of coronal tissue damage relative to the pulp chamber, root/canal morphology, and alveolar bone levels
- pulp sensibility/vitality
- an occlusal analysis to ascertain the loading, guidance, or interferences that may be related to the tooth in question, in all axes of movement
- occlusal vertical dimension (OVD) assessment to ensure that there is enough inter-occlusal space to place a restoration successfully. Tilting/over-eruption of the tooth or opposing teeth may reduce the space available in which to place a secure restoration with adequate strength, so forcing treatment down the more complex reorganized approach to dental rehabilitation (see Chapter 5, Section 5.14).

When considering the tooth to be restored itself, further factors to consider would include the following:

- *Amount/distribution of the remaining viable tooth structure.* In posterior teeth, the presence of solid cusps directly or diagonally opposite one another can help to support and even retain the core restoration with relative undercuts (see later). On the other hand, thin, weaker retained buccal or lingual/palatal walls would be less amenable to preparation for the retention of amalgam, and more prone to fracture. In these situations, the retained, weaker cusps/walls may be reduced in height vertically and the core material overlaid to offer some occlusal loading pressure relief during function (see Figure 6.1). When placing adhesive resin composite cores, care must be taken to limit shrinkage stresses at the tooth–restoration interface using incremental techniques and when considering the axial tooth preparation that might be required for the indirect crown to be fitted.
- *The sub-gingival extent of the coronal damage.* When fragments of tooth–restoration complex have been lost in function, the fractures

Table 6.1 General clinical factors to be considered when deciding whether a broken down tooth is restorable or not in a particular patient

Factor	Favourable	Less favourable
Pulp	Vital pulp with adequate RDT to incorporate tooth preparation	Symptoms present, PA pathology (RCT will be required; isolation/access cavity compromised?)
RCT status	Good-quality sealed RCT, assessed radiographically with PA resolution evident. Straight canals and broad roots facilitate post placement	Symptomatic, recurrence of PA pathology, re-RCT required? Thin roots and curved canals prevent post placement
Tooth structure	Adequate bulk remaining (e.g. cusps) Adequate distribution of coronal tissues. No cracks/defects	Inadequate quantities available once tooth preparation has occurred leads to weakness and fracture
Existing restoration status	Only requires refurbishment or repair (see Chapter 9)	Active caries present, leaking margins, subgingival extension
Periodontal status	Pocket depths 3–4 mm, minimal recession, > 50% bone level from PA radiographs	Active periodontal disease, LOA, < 50% bone levels, grade II–III mobility
Occlusion Dental arch tooth position	Protected canine guided lateral excursions. No interferences Fully/partially dentate with even tooth distribution, minimal tilting/rotations	Reduced OVD minimizes space for restoration Tooth bears full occlusal load in a quadrant, drifted/tilted/rotated
Aesthetics	Posterior dentition, previously restored dentition	High smile line in anterior aesthetic zone, recession risk due to thin gingival tissues, subgingival restoration margins, and poor contour; complex shade matching
Patient factors: preventive status	Well-motivated responsible patient, efficacious oral hygiene control (or can be educated to be such)	Refuses to take responsibility for/unable to maintain oral health; poor diet, oral hygiene, no fluoride use

RDT, remaining dentine thickness; RCT, root canal treatment; PA, periapical; LOA, loss of attachment; OVD, occlusal vertical dimension.

that occur often follow natural internal histological planes, leading to shear fractures that can terminate on the root surface several millimetres subgingivally (see Figure 6.2). This makes their restoration difficult in terms of preparing the subsequent base cavity form to support the core restoration as well as gaining direct access and moisture control, thus adversely affecting the successful medium- to long-term restorability of the tooth.

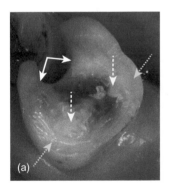 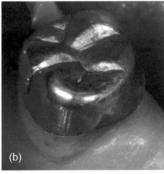

Figure 6.1 (a) A heavily broken down mandibular molar. The original mesial-occlusal-distal (MOD) amalgam cavity has been modified macro-mechanically to aid retention and support of the larger core restoration to be placed. The white arrows show the relative proximal undercut in the distal box. The green dotted arrows indicate how the thinner, weaker mesiobuccal cusp and lingual walls have been reduced in occlusal height and prepared with a shoulder finish to support the new overlaid amalgam restoration margin (and be protected by it). The yellow dashed arrows show retentive grooves which have been cut into the healthy dentine (avoiding the pulp chamber), into which amalgam will be packed. **(b)** The large amalgam core restoration after several years of function. (Courtesy of L. Mackenzie.)

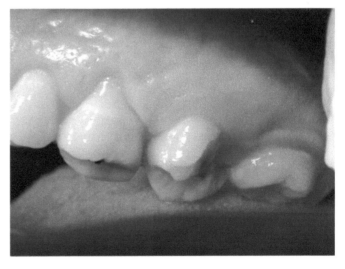

Figure 6.2 A mirror image of the UR5, 6, 7, 8, showing a traumatic distal shear fracture of the still vital UR7 terminating subgingivally on the root surface.

Q6.1: What practical difficulties might be encountered when trying to restore the tooth shown in Figure 6.2?

- *Using the pulp and/or root canal spaces.* If the tooth has undergone successful root canal treatment (RCT), there is the potential to prepare the straight portion of a root canal for a post, which can then help to retain the core restoration (see Figure 6.4). Restorative core material can fill the pulp chamber and even the first 2–3 mm of root canal space, close to the orifice, so gaining mechanical retention. When this type of restoration, originally using amalgam, is placed, it is known as a 'Nayyar core' (see Chapter 7, Section 7.5.3 and Chapter 8, Section 8.10). With the development of modern, high-quality adhesive dental restorative materials to aid core retention, the need for elective RCT of a vital tooth for core retention is not normally indicated.

- *The direct core restorative material.* The traditional restorative material used for core restorations, especially on posterior teeth, is dental amalgam, due to its high compressive strength and wear resistance under occlusal loading. Contemporary resin composites have an improved strength and wear resistance compared with their predecessors, and as they will often be covered with an indirect crown, these are now becoming more popular as core materials (see Figure 6.4e). Their adhesive retention properties reduce the amount of tooth preparation required, making them an attractive proposition where remaining tooth structure is at a premium (see Chapter 5, Section 5.10). However, moisture control and the relative complexity of their placement technique in multiple increments in cavities that are not always easy to access operatively or keep dry can limit their use successfully in this regard.

6.3 Intra-coronal core restoration

The key functions of the direct plastic core restoration used to build up the broken down tooth include:

- reconstituting the structure, function, and possibly the aesthetics of the crown of the tooth

- maintaining pulp vitality, or where a RCT is present, ensuring that the coronal endodontic seal is maintained

- providing indirect support, stability, and retention for the overlying indirect laboratory-made restoration, if required

- de-bulking/reducing the volume of the more expensive overlying indirect restoration—this will be more relevant when precious metals are used in its construction.

The direct core restoration is in the form of a plastic restorative material (e.g. amalgam, resin composite). However, in some cases, depending on the distribution and quantity of remaining tooth structure and the size and shape of the existing cavity, an indirect/cast inlay/onlay or partial crown restoration may be placed instead of the plastic core build-up. Materials used for this type of restoration would include indirect resin composite, precious and non-precious metal alloys, or ceramics.

6.3.1 Direct core retention

The retention mechanisms used for different plastic restorative materials have been highlighted in Table 5.8 in Chapter 5. *Macro-mechanical* cavity modifications to aid restoration retention will include the provision of diametrically opposing hard tissue undercuts where possible, without over-preparing and weakening the remaining tooth structure unnecessarily. Opposing surfaces can be made more plane parallel with marginal shoulder preparations to stabilize the final restoration, and minimally invasive stabilizing slots and grooves can be placed within healthy tissues where possible (see Figure 6.3).

C factor

Adhesive materials will be placed with suitable bonding systems (see Table 8.12 in Chapter 8). Incremental layering techniques must be used for conventional resin composite materials. This minimizes the polymerization shrinkage stresses concentrating at the tooth–restoration interface which can lead to potential tooth flexure and even cracks, with concomitant symptoms of sensitivity. However, in large open cavities with a reduced ratio of bonded surface area to free surface area (the C factor), the shrinkage stresses will be less problematic.

- An occlusal cavity with a ratio of five bonded surfaces to one unbonded surface has the highest C factor, of 5 (i.e. 5:1), thus maximizing the interfacial stresses.

- A labial resin composite veneer has the lowest C factor, of 1 (a ratio of one bonded to one free surface, both of similar surface area). In this case, the shrinkage (on average in the range 1.5–2.5% by volume for many modern resin composites) will be dissipated within the restoration and not concentrated at the tooth–restoration interface (see Figures 6.4d and 6.4e).

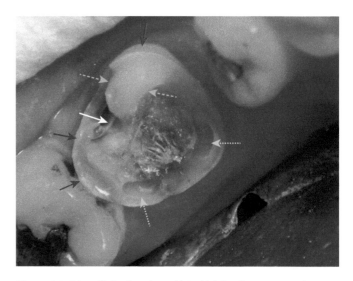

Figure 6.3 A heavily broken down LL6 which has been prepared macromechanically to receive an amalgam core restoration. The blue dashed arrows indicate the relative undercut prepared around the vertically reduced mesiobuccal cusp, which will be overlaid with amalgam. The green dotted arrows point to two slots that have been prepared in healthy dentine to aid retention of the amalgam. The small purple arrows highlight the prepared distal-buccal shoulder to support the amalgam restoration margin. The amalgam placement procedure is described in detail in Chapter 8, Section 8.9. (Courtesy of G. Palmer.)

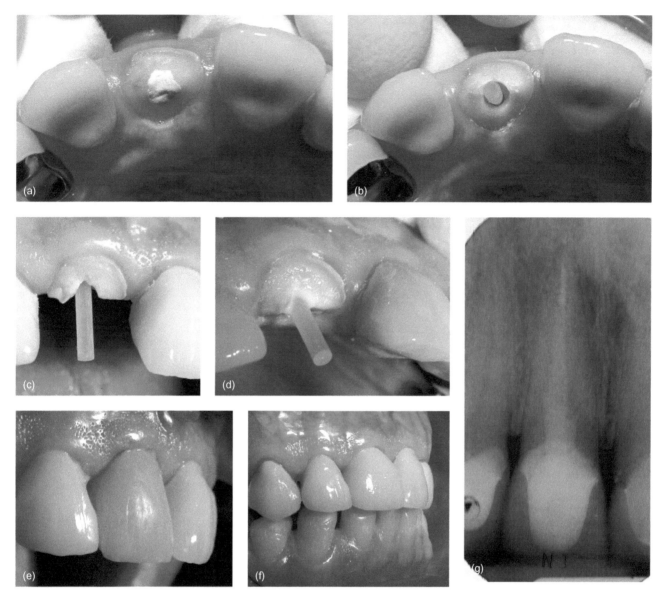

Figure 6.4 (a) Fractured UR1. The crown fractured through the pulp chamber during mastication. The remaining root was endodontically treated and a temporary restoration was placed in the access cavity. The fracture margins are just at the gingival margin or supragingival. The remaining enamel and dentine are sound. **(b)** and **(c)** show the root canal post space having been created using increasing sizes of Gate Glidden burs. A fibre-reinforced direct post has been placed into the post space. Its length has been adjusted to ensure that it is short of the incisal edge position of the final restoration. **(d)** The fibre-reinforced post has been cemented into the canal space using a resin cement, and the excess has been removed before final photo-curing. **(e)** Direct provisional resin composite restoration built up incrementally around the fibre post. **(f)** Definitive indirect ceramic cast restoration UR1 in occlusion. **(g)** Final periapical radiograph showing the fibre-reinforced post in place with 4 mm of root canal filling material (gutta-percha) still present at the apical end of the root canal. Note the similar radiodensity of the fibre post compared with the surrounding dentine.

Q6.2:

i Look at Figure 6.4 (a). What other restorative materials could be used to fill the endodontic access cavity?

ii Look at Figure 6.4 (b). Why should the post diameter not exceed one-third of the root diameter?

iii Look at Figure 6.4 (c). Why should the post extend to 1–2 mm below the incisal edge/occlusal surface of the definitive restoration?

iv Look at Figure 6.4 (d). Can you suggest any alternative materials used to cement a root canal post?

v Look at Figure 6.4 (e). What is the C factor of this provisional restoration?

vi Look at Figure 6.4 (f). Why should the post length within the root canal exceed the length of the final restoration it supports?

To date, there is limited independent published evidence to validate the use of bulk-fill resin composites, which only need one large increment of material to fill a larger cavity, as a core restorative material (see Chapter 7, Section 7.2.2). However, this class of resin composite is popular among dentists due to its simplicity of use and—anecdotally at present—these materials seem to offer at least medium-term success. High-viscosity glass ionomer cements and their derivatives have been used as core materials, but as a general rule these materials are not recommended routinely for this purpose unless there are at least two opposing walls of tooth tissue present. Their only moderate compressive strength and wear resistance, when compared with amalgam and resin composites, also makes them less appropriate for use as long-lasting restorations exposed to extensive occlusal functional loading.

In the restoration of endodontically treated teeth, the cementation of a post into the root canal space is indicated if the amount of residual tooth structure is insufficient to support a core made of a plastic material (amalgam or resin composite). The roots must also have sufficient bulk (diameter), and must have a length of straight root canal longer than the height of the final restoration it will support. Root canal posts require removal of the root canal filling material (often gutta-percha) within the coronal two-thirds of a straight canal. The procedure usually commences with a small rose head bur in a slow-speed handpiece, then continuing with a specially designed steel Gates Glidden bur. This consists of a non-cutting point on the end, which melts the gutta-percha, and then a bulbous cutting tip with a narrow shank behind that allows the root filling material to be spun out of the canal space—all in one action. The coronal root canal space then needs to be increased in size to accommodate a post. This is achieved with a special twist drill (often supplied with the post kit) mounted in the slow-speed handpiece, shaped to match the size of post selected. The maximum width of the post is normally equal to one-third of the diameter of the remaining root, assessed from the periapical radiograph. There should be at least 4 mm of residual root canal filling material remaining at the root apex, to ensure that the existing apical endodontic seal is not disturbed. All of these dimensions can be assessed from the preoperative periapical radiograph (see Figure 6.4).

6.4 Clinical operative tips

- The ability to achieve successful moisture control is critical to the ultimate long-term restorability of the broken down tooth. Clamping the individual tooth for rubber dam placement may not be possible due to the scarcity of supra-gingival tooth structure. A split-dam technique may be required, with the dam anchored to adjacent teeth and the use of circumferential floss ligatures around the broken down tooth, to adapt the dam to the tooth to be restored (see Section 5.6.3).

- In some cases, the use of cotton wool rolls/judicious suction may be all that is possible in this regard (see Section 5.6.2).

- Historically, a suitably adapted copper ring or, if available, an orthodontic band can be used to support the core restoration build-up circumferentially, and retained while the restorative material sets in function, before its removal at a subsequent visit.

- Attempt to make internal cavity walls as plane parallel or slightly undercut as required without the concomitant loss of unnecessary sound tooth structure. Opposing walls help the stability of the core restoration within the cavity (see Figures 6.1a and 6.4).

- Careful use of slots, grooves, and pits can help the retention of large core restorations (see Figure 6.1a and 6.4).

- *Matrixing:* Various designs of circumferential matrix exist, ranging from copper/orthodontic bands to self-tightening and supporting auto-matrix systems (see Chapter 5, Section 5.12). These are most useful for aiding the build-up of multiple missing walls of large cavities. Problems commonly arise when there is little peripheral tooth structure to support the outline shape of the band and, on tightening, the band collapses over, especially where extensive cusps and walls are missing, resulting in open proximal contacts and poor final restoration morphology.

Clinical techniques to overcome this loss of restoration morphology and contact points include the following:

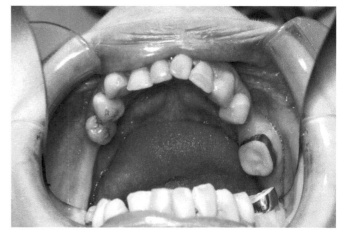

Figure 6.5 A mirror view of a stainless steel orthodontic band placed around the LL6, supporting a large coronal restoration following endodontic treatment and prior to provision of an indirect full-coverage restoration. Note how the band has been adapted well to the contour of the molar and burnished into the furcation defect buccally. Regarding the clinical photography, note the use of cheek retractors and an occlusal mirror which is kept demisted by first heating it up in warm water prior to drying it and using it intra-orally. It is then subjected to a gentle air stream from the 3-1 syringe by the nurse who holds the mirror steady. The patient can hold the retractors once positioned by the operator.

Q6.3: What clinical clues in the patient shown in Figure 6.5 might help you gain an insight into the patient's high caries risk, prior to when the image was taken?

- Trimming/shaping the outline of the matrix band to help proximal placement through tight contact points, adaptation, and contour of the restoration.
- Using a ball burnisher hand instrument (see Figure 5.26 in Chapter 5), burnish the matrix band once in place, tightened and wedged proximally to adapt the band to the cervical margin of the tooth.
- Tightening and wedging the band proximally, filling the depth of the proximal boxes with initial small increments of restorative material (e.g. flowable resin composite). Then loosening the matrix a little to adjust its position and allow burnishing adaptation at the contact point, followed by further increments of material. This 'adaptive matrixing' permits close adaptation at the cavity floor and adequate contouring of the proximal restoration anatomy.
- Initially restore the accessible cusps, lingual/palatal, and buccal/labial walls without the aid of a matrix band. Once restored, place the matrix band conventionally (circumferential or sectional), wedge and restore the proximal areas to the correct contact point and proximal morphology.
- The clinical procedure for placing a fibre-reinforced post and building up a resin composite core is outlined in Table 8.11 in Chapter 8. Endodontically restored teeth may need endodontic re-treatments, and in this respect well-bonded fibre posts can be removed, but considerable care is needed. Their removal is achieved by drilling down through the middle of the post, avoiding any additional removal of peripheral root or coronal dentine. In contrast, removal of a non-adhesively cemented metal-based post may be relatively easy, using an ultrasonic scaler to break down the cement at the post–dentine interface. Unfortunately, an adhesively cemented metal post will be nearly impossible to remove without damaging the remaining root dentine.

6.5 Design principles for indirect restorations

This section aims to *outline* the common design features required for the successful placement of indirect laboratory or chair-side made restorations used to reconstruct the crowns of broken down teeth. It does not cover the details of specific individual step-by-step restoration preparations, materials, or operative techniques involved in the clinical and laboratory manufacturing process. This information is available in alternative prosthodontic texts.

Indirect restorations are classified as those that are fabricated outside the mouth—either by dentists making temporary crowns from putty indices, or technicians making restorations in a dental laboratory or from a clinical CAD-CAM processing unit from intra-oral records—and then cemented into place clinically by the operator (see Table 6.2). They may be appropriate in the following clinical situations:

- to protect a broken down, weakened tooth from further fracture or to hold together parts of a cracked tooth (cusps, walls)
- to restore an already broken tooth or a tooth that has been severely worn down
- to cover, support, and protect a tooth with an extensive core restoration from large occlusal loads when there is little tooth structure remaining
- to retain a bridge, whose *pontic(s)* replace the missing tooth/teeth and *abutments* anchor the prosthesis to adjacent tooth/teeth
- to cover severely misshapen or discoloured teeth where direct restorative methods would not be clinically or practically viable

Table 6.2 The different designs of indirect restorations and the range of materials used to manufacture them. The intrinsic properties of the materials, often needing to be optimal in thin section, will include a combination of suitable compressive, shear, and tensile strengths (to combat occlusal loading), wear resistance (ideally comparable to enamel), and aesthetics

Indirect restoration type	Materials
Inlay	Gold type I alloy, ceramic, laboratory composite
Onlay	Gold type II and III alloy, composite, ceramic
Partial coverage crown (e.g. three-quarter crown)	Gold type III alloy
Full coverage crown (full gold crown (FGC), metal ceramic crown (MCC)/porcelain-fused-to-metal crown (PFM), all-ceramic crowns)	Gold type III alloy, palladium alloy, base metal alloys (nickel, chromium), ceramic, stainless steel (paediatric crowns)
Precision attachments	Gold type III and IV alloy, palladium or base metal alloy (nickel, chromium)
Temporary crowns	Acrylate resin/acrylic based

- to restore dental implant abutments and to act as precision attachments for removable prostheses.

For children, an indirect crown may be used on the primary dentition in order to:

- save a tooth that has been so damaged by caries that it can longer support a filling, but requires maintenance in the dental arch for functional and developmental reasons (the Hall technique)
- protect the teeth of a child at high risk for caries, especially if he or she has difficulty maintaining daily oral hygiene
- decrease the frequency of sedation and general anaesthesia for children who are unable because of age, behaviour, or medical history to fully cooperate with the requirements of proper dental care/maintenance.

In such cases, a paediatric dentist is likely to recommend a stainless steel crown.

6.5.1 Design features

Retention is the property of a restoration/cavity that prevents its displacement from the cavity in its direction of placement/insertion. Prior to the use of chemical adhesives, this property was reliant on macro-mechanical tooth preparation features, including undercuts (only for direct plastic restorations), slots, and grooves, which potentially weakened and sacrificed quantities of sound tooth structure (see Chapter 5, Section 5.10).

Resistance form is the property of a restoration/cavity that prevents its displacement in any other direction.

These traditional terms have gone out of fashion somewhat, and indeed their use was always rather more theoretical than practical. Their relevance is much reduced in contemporary minimally invasive operative dentistry since the advent and development of dental adhesives. However, basic mechanical principles are still relevant and important when designing preparations suitable for indirect restorations of all types of material:

- *Occlusal/axial reduction.* This should be sufficient to accommodate the appropriate thickness of restorative material used for the indirect restoration. Gold alloy crowns require the least tooth preparation, as they have adequate strength/ rigidity in thin section (0.7 mm). Indirect resin composites and all-ceramic restorations require a greater bulk (up to 2 mm) to achieve this. Newer ceramic formulations allow thinner veneers with adequate strength and aesthetics, so making tooth preparation more minimally invasive.
- *Axial wall taper (see Figure 6.6a and b).* For indirect restorations that have been manufactured and cast or cured outside the mouth, perfectly parallel walls would be ideal, but in practice these are impossible to achieve without introducing an element of undercut. Instead, a slightly divergent axial taper of 7–10 degrees is recommended. Even this level of taper is difficult to achieve/perceive with the naked eye in the oral cavity; therefore 15 degrees is often the minimum achieved in practice. Any undercut in the axial surface preparation (as with classic amalgam cavities, see Chapter 5, Section 5.10, Figures 5.48 and 5.49) is contraindicated, as it will be impossible to make or seat the restoration.
- *Surface area and finish.* Maximizing the surface area between the indirect restoration and tooth will aid cementation and therefore

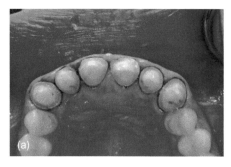
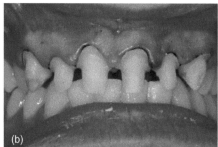
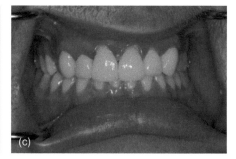

Figure 6.6 **(a)** A maxillary anterior occlusal view of full coverage indirect crown preparations, UR3-UL3. Note the supragingival location of the rounded shoulder finishing margins of the tapered axial walls. **(b)** The labial view of the same tooth preparations where the rounded shoulder finishing margins are more clearly demarcated, as is their circumferential position supragingival to the surrounding gingival papillae. The relative tapering of the axial walls can be clearly seen on the upper central incisor teeth. Sufficient occlusal height reduction of the teeth allows **(c)** the final ceramic restorations to be cemented using a resin-based luting cement. (Courtesy of Dr Ryan Olley.)

Q6.4:

i   What are the advantages and disadvantages of placing the axial wall finishing margins supragingivally as shown in Figure 6.6 (a)?

ii Do you know what the black lines are adjacent to the finishing margins of the six prepared teeth as shown in Figure 6.6 (b)?

retention. The microscopic surface produced by fine dental diamond/tungsten carbon finishing burs will increase the surface area for adhesive bonding without introducing major flaws or cracks in the tooth tissue (see Chapter 5, Sections 5.82 and 5.83).

- *Preparation margin (see Figure 6.6a and b): position.* To maximize the axial wall length and surface area, it is desirable to place the finishing margin of the full coverage crown close to but just supragingival. This will aid oral hygiene procedures for the patient and allow simpler impression taking for the operator. Care must be taken during tooth preparation not to traumatize the gingival tissues or to encroach on the biologic width of the gingival attachment complex (the region between the alveolar bone crest and junctional epithelial attachment), for fear of accelerating irreversible periodontal tissue damage and recession. The patient must be advised about optimal oral hygiene procedures to prevent plaque biofilm stagnation at the restoration margins. Indeed, if a patient shows evidence of not being able to maintain suitable oral hygiene around such areas, this should potentially act as a contraindication to restoration placement (see Table 6.1).

- *Preparation margin: shape.* The cross-sectional shape of the margin between indirect restoration and tooth should be a *chamfer* or a *rounded shoulder* configuration. This is dependent on the following:

  - The type of material used to fabricate the restoration. Gold and other metal alloy margins can be manufactured to finer tolerances, so reducing the amount of tooth preparation required at the interface between restoration and tooth. Ceramics require a greater bulk of material for strength and aesthetics, resulting in heavier marginal tooth preparation (see Figures 6.6c and 6.7).

  - The amount of tooth structure/core restoration present. The most tooth-preserving, minimally invasive margin preparation is a minimal chamfered finish, which may be desirable where remaining tooth structure is at a premium and not easily accessible.

  - The position of the margin. When lingual, distal, or palatal, margins can be finished in metal without an aesthetic compromise, so needing only a minimally invasive chamfer finish. Indeed, cir-

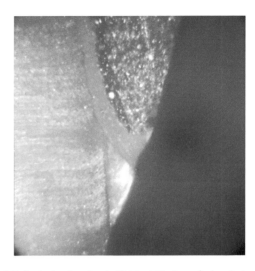

Figure 6.7 A photomicrograph (field width 2 mm) showing a section through the margin interface of a thin ceramic restoration luted to a tooth. The dentine is on the left of the image, and the ceramic restoration is on the upper right. Between it and the dentine and the small triangle of retained enamel is the resin-based luting cement. The profile of the axial finishing margin on the tooth is a chamfer.

cumferential indirect restoration margins may have different configurations dependent upon their anatomical position (labial vs. proximal vs. lingual/palatal).

The different margin configurations are prepared using end-cutting burs with a rounded tip (half depth) to achieve a chamfer (see Figure 6.7), and a squared off tip profile to achieve a shoulder.

- *Adhesive resin cement.* Modern adhesive cements have chemical moieties that can bond to ions in the tooth as well as oxides and other chemical groups within the restorative material, so providing some chemical adhesion (see Figure 6.7). This permits greater leeway in the mechanical accuracy of the tooth preparation (including the degree of taper of the axial walls, their surface finish, and surface area).

6.6 Answers to self-test questions

Q6.1: What practical difficulties might be encountered when trying to restore the tooth shown in Figure 6.2?

A:

i Difficult physical instrument access to the distal of the UR7.

ii Difficult moisture control (hard to place rubber dam).

iii Difficult to modify cavity form at the base of the shear fracture.

iv Difficult to place restorative material at base of fracture (adhesive or otherwise). A possible solution to improving the restorability of the tooth would be to carry out a crown-lengthening procedure to relocate the gingival margin apically, so improving access to the base of the cavity.

Q6.2:

i Look at Figure 6.4 (a). What other restorative materials could be used to fill the endodontic access cavity?

A: GIC, resin composite.

ii Look at Figure 6.4 (b). Why should the post diameter not exceed one-third of the root diameter?

A: If the post is wider than this ratio, there is an increased risk of root fracture, especially with metal-based posts which do not dissipate stresses evenly through the root length.

iii Look at Figure 6.4 (c). Why should the post extend to 1–2 mm below the incisal edge/occlusal surface of the definitive restoration?

A: So that there is enough space afforded to the core restoration to cover the post. When the core restoration is prepared for a crown, up to 2 mm of clearance may be needed occlusally/incisally. There is a risk that the post may be exposed during crown preparation, and this can potentially weaken the core structure or even the fibre post.

iv Look at Figure 6.4 (d). Can you suggest any alternative materials used to cement a root canal post?

A: GIC-based cements.

v Look at Figure 6.4 (e). What is the C factor of this provisional restoration?

A: The C factor is calculated as the ratio of the bonded surface area to the dentine vs. the non-bonded surface of the resin composite restoration. As you can see from the series of images, the bonded surface is small compared with the rest of the restoration, so this is a favourable configuration. Thus stress concentrations at the interface will be minimal.

vi Look at Figure 6.4 (g). Why should the post length within the root canal exceed the length of the final restoration it supports?

A: Mechanically, this provides the best distribution of occlusal loading forces on the post–restoration–tooth complex. If the post length is shorter than its supported restoration, unfavourable fulcrums of force can be generated, leading to crown or root fracture in clinical use.

Q6.3: What clinical clues in the patient shown in Figure 6.5 might help you gain an insight into the patient's high caries risk, prior to when the image was taken?

A: The presence, site, and number of tooth-coloured adhesive restorations and the apparently untreated buccal carious lesion on the LR5.

Q6.4:

i What are the advantages and disadvantages of placing the axial wall finishing margins supragingivally as shown in Figure 6.6 (a)?

A: Advantages: no trauma to the gingiva during preparation; easier recording of margins in the final impression; easier to construct accurate temporary crowns; easier for the laboratory to fabricate accurately fitting crowns; less likelihood of the periodontium being adversely affected and thereby leading to later recession or periodontal disease; easier for the patient to clean the restoration margins. Disadvantages: anteriorly, aesthetics may be compromised as the margins may be visible in a patient with a high lip line.

ii Do you know what the black lines are adjacent to the finishing margins of the six prepared teeth as shown in Figure 6.6 (b)?

A: Gingival retraction cord placed carefully into the periodontal pocket, to help to keep the gingival tissue away from the tooth during impression taking. It helps to dry the field and stops bleeding, especially if the margins are subgingival (due to the astringent in which the cord is soaked).

7

Restorative materials and their relationship to tooth structure

Chapter contents

7.1 Introduction

Modern restorative materials can be classified in several ways, in terms of their retention (chemically adhesive, macro-, micro- or even nano-mechanical), their chemistry (e.g. resin-based vs. acid–base reaction, filler particles), or their clinical properties (e.g. aesthetics, strength, handling). It is essential that these materials are considered closely with the histological substrate to which they will adhere or with which they will interact, in order to understand the complexities of each system and their potential clinical uses.

This chapter will outline and discuss aspects of dental materials science to enable the reader to understand and appreciate the links with relevant histology and relate this to the clinical aspects of minimally invasive operative dentistry. Also discussed is dental amalgam, still a popular restorative material among many dentists worldwide, although clinical indications for its use are becoming more limited as treatment rationales change and adhesive materials improve. This text will require supplementation from suitable dental histology and detailed dental material science texts.

7.2 Dental resin composite

Dental resin composites are aesthetic, plastic adhesive restorative materials that consist of co-polymerized methacrylate-based resin chains embedding inert filler particles (conferring strength and wear resistance) and requiring a separate adhesive (bonding agent) to micro-/nano-mechanically bond them to either enamel or dentine, respectively. However, not all modern dental composites are based purely on this methacrylate resin chemistry (see Section 7.2.6). Therefore the term 'composite resin' is inappropriate and should not be used.

7.2.1 History

Resin composites have developed over the past 50 years, after the introduction of the acid-etch technique (Buonocore, 1955) and methacrylate monomers (Bowen's resin—Bis-GMA (1971); see Section 7.2.2).

7.2.2 Chemistry

Methacrylate resins

The unset (or uncured) material consists of a mixture of several different types of resin methacrylate monomers, most of which are hydrophobic (water-hating) in nature (see Figure 7.1).

The monomer chain length affects certain properties of the resin composite:

- *Viscosity (or flowability) of the material.* This is important in order to minimize voids trapped within the uncured composite during placement and packing within the depths of a cavity (the stiffer the consistency, the greater the risk of trapping air voids). The shorter the uncured monomer length (and therefore the lower the molecular weight), the lower is its viscosity. Often shorter-length, lower-molecular-weight methacrylate monomers form the basis of the resin chemistry of flowable resin composites, and other diluent molecules may be added.

- *Volumetric polymerization shrinkage of composite on curing.* The setting process is a light-activated, free-radical addition polymerization chain reaction. The shorter the monomer chains, the more of them need to join per unit volume, and the increased reduction in space between them leads to the relatively increased shrinkage exhibited (1.5–3.5% by volume; see Figure 7.2).

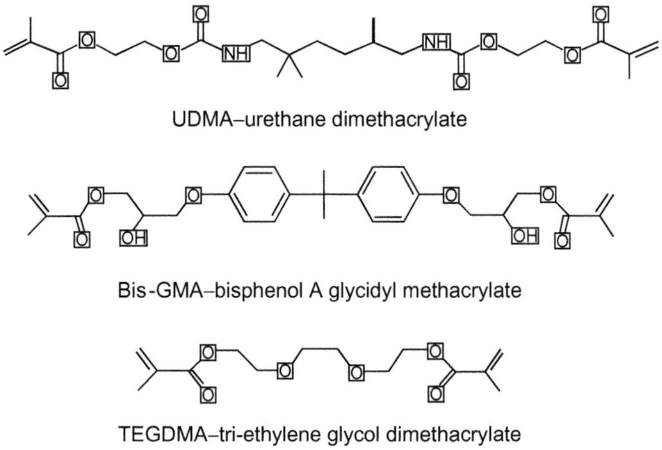

UDMA–urethane dimethacrylate

Bis-GMA–bisphenol A glycidyl methacrylate

TEGDMA–tri-ethylene glycol dimethacrylate

Figure 7.1 Examples with chemical formulae of methacrylate resins commonly used in dental composites. Note how TEGDMA has a shorter chain length than the others.

Q7.1: What properties of the resin composite are affected by monomer chain length?

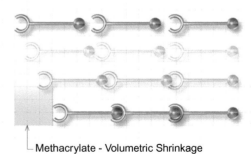

Methacrylate - Volumetric Shrinkage

Figure 7.2 A diagrammatic representation of linear monomers undergoing addition polymerization leading to volumetric shrinkage. (Courtesy of 3M ESPE.)

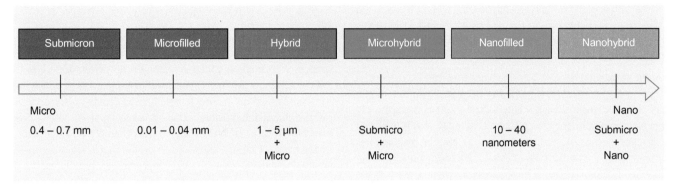

Figure 7.3 A table showing the size ranges of filler particles in a range of modern resin composites. (Courtesy of Septodont UK.)

Filler particles

See Figure 7.3. Inert filler particles are made from silica, quartz, barium, or strontium glass derivatives (introducing radio-opacity), and are embedded in and bound to the resin matrix using a coating of an organo-silane coupling agent (γ-methacryloxypropyltrimethoxysilane (γ-MPTS)). Over the past 40 years, manufacturers have attempted to pack in various sizes/shapes of particle in increasing numbers per unit volume in an effort to improve the clinical properties of resin composites. The more space that is taken up by irregular and spherical-shaped filler particles, the less space there is for native resin monomer, leading to a reduction in overall shrinkage on curing. Conversely, the more filler particles that are loaded into the composite, the more viscous it becomes, so there is a fine balance to be struck between the filler load and its resin content. The filler particles confer several properties on the cured composite material:

- *Wear characteristics*: increasing the density of larger, harder, and more irregular shaped filler particles will tend to increase the wear resistance of the composite, as less resin matrix will be exposed at the restoration surface.

- *Surface polish*: the smaller, softer, and more spherical-shaped the filler particles, the more polishable (but also less wear resistant) the resin composite.

- *Aesthetics*: the finer the filler particles, the more aesthetic the composite, as the optical properties can be made to match more accurately those of enamel. Modern resin composites can have numerous shades (using pigments and various degrees of opacity) or just a few, relying on a 'chameleon' effect where a relatively translucent resin composite can encompass several tooth shades, blending into the surrounding natural colours very effectively by transmitting colour from them.

- *Physical properties (e.g. compressive and shear strength, elasticity)*: the correct balance between filler particle and resin content is required to ensure optimal physical properties.

Other chemical ingredients

These small fractions include *inhibitors* (butyl-4-hydroxytoluenes (BHT), to increase material longevity prior to curing), *photo-initiators* (see later), *accelerators* (dimethylaminobenzoates (DMAB), to increase the reactivity of the photo-initiator, thereby speeding up curing time), *photo-stabilizers* (2-hydroxy-4-methoxybenzophenone (HMBP), to provide colour stability by eliminating UV action on amine initiators), *radio-opacifiers* (aluminium, titanium, or zirconium oxides), and *colour pigments* (various ferric and titanium oxides).

Setting reaction

The setting (curing) process in modern resin composites is either light-activated (470 nm wavelength visible blue light) or dual-cured, light and chemical activation (initiated by 0.5% benzoyl peroxide and activated using dimethyl-p-toluidine). Light-cured resin composite contains a photo-initiator, α-diketone (camphorquinone) and an amine, which under the activation of visible blue light generates the free radicals required to initiate the cross-linking polymerization chain reaction. Some issues related to the setting reaction of resins include the following:

- *Low degree of monomer conversion (50–77%)*: not all of the free monomer polymerizes on curing, leaving some to leach out of the composite, so contributing to the long-term degradation of the material in terms of moisture ingress and possible sensitization issues with some patients.

- *High linear/volumetric shrinkage on curing (1.5–3.5%)*: Figure 7.2 illustrates how shrinkage occurs during polymerization and leads to the composite pulling away from cavity margins, so increasing the risk of marginal leakage.

- *High shrinkage stress at the composite–tooth interface (3–8 MPa)*: the stresses generated by the polymerization process can be high at cavity margins, depending on the cavity C factor (the ratio of bonded to unbonded surfaces; see Chapter 6), the bulk of the material, and the compliance of the cavity walls. This can lead to debonding and tooth fracture of the weakened marginal tissues.

- *Water absorption*: water is absorbed hygroscopically during and after the curing process, leading to expansion, long-term composite degradation, and staining.

- *Air-inhibited surface layer of uncured resin*: the free-radical addition polymerization reaction is inhibited by air. After curing an increment of resin composite material, a glossy film of uncured resin is retained on the surface of the composite, and the monomers in this layer are used to provide adherence for the next increment placed upon it. In this way, resin composite can be added to within a cavity to build up the final restoration.

- *Depth of cure*: conventional resin composites can be cured to a depth of 2–3 mm (depending on the translucency of the material). A thicker section will not cure sufficiently at its base (the 470 nm light does not penetrate sufficiently at those depths to permit activation of the polymerization reaction), and the resulting restoration may then be described as having a 'soggy bottom.' Note that resin composites cure most efficiently when closest to the 470 nm light source, which must be placed as close as possible to the uncured composite and should be built up in small angled increments.

- *'Bulk fill' resin composites:* these materials are promoted by certain manufacturers as being suitable for use as a dentine replacement in the restoration of large deep cavities. They are usually of a relatively low-viscosity, 'flowable' consistency so that they will achieve good adaptation to the cavity floor and walls, almost 'self-levelling' within the cavity. Mechanical properties, such as toughness, will be reduced to achieve this effect, but this may be an acceptable compromise within the depths of a large cavity. Their depth of cure is achieved by the use of a relatively transparent material, often with large filler particles, so allowing good light transmission and hence monomer conversion. There are also more viscous, heavily filled versions of these materials, which can be placed in bulk, but there are compromises in their handling, such as achieving adequate adaptation on the cavity floor (leading to voids), good contact points, and the development of occlusal anatomy.

7.2.3 The tooth–resin composite interface

Table 7.1 highlights some of the clinically important histological features of sound enamel and dentine relevant to the restoration of tooth surfaces with modern adhesive materials. An understanding of the interactions between the chemistry of the materials and this relevant histology is vital in order to optimize the qualities of the adhesive restorative systems available, including resin composites. Table 7.2 outlines the clinical properties that each layer of dental hard tissue confers on the crown of a tooth, and those properties that a restorative material should exhibit to act as an ideal replacement material for each.

Resin composite and enamel

Hydrophobic resin composites adhere to dry enamel micro-mechanically, and the prismatic, crystalline ultrastructure of enamel permits this to happen successfully, reliably, and strongly (20–50 MPa bond strengths have been measured in laboratory studies). Three stages are required to develop the bond between resin composite and enamel after the enamel has been prepared mechanically during cavity preparation:

1. Acid etching (alternative US term is 'conditioning')—this is the process of placing 37% orthophosphoric acid gel on to the prepared enamel surface for 20 seconds. This:

   - removes surface contaminants (saliva, proteinaceous substances) and the smear layer (a tenacious surface layer of organic and inorganic cutting debris < 20 μm thick) and increases the surface area for bonding

   - produces micro-irregularities/micro-porosities in the prismatic enamel surface. This microscopic surface roughness will provide micro-mechanical retention for the resin (see Figure 7.4).

Table 7.1 Clinically relevant histology that interacts with the chemistry of modern adhesive restorative materials

	Mineral (inorganic)	Matrix (organic)	Structural arrangement
Enamel	Calcium hydroxyapatite crystallites $(Ca_{10}(PO_4)_7(OH)_2$: $40 \times 70 \times 170$ nm) 97% by weight, 89% by volume	No collagen Enamelins (MW 55 kDa), amelogenins (MW 25 kDa): 1% by weight, 2% by volume Water: 3% by weight, 9% by volume	10 000 crystallites arranged into *prisms* (US-rods); EDJ to surface; ameloblasts—Tomes' processes; 4–7 μm diameter; undulation, decussation; keyhole pattern in cross-section; prism cores/boundaries exist due to change in orientation of crystallites Aprismatic layer at tooth surface on eruption
Dentine	Calcium hydroxyapatite crystallites (with Mg and CO_3 substitutions: $5 \times 30 \times 80$ nm) β-octocalcium phosphate crystals	90% collagen: Type I $([\alpha1(I)]_2\alpha2(I))$ with trace amounts of type I trimer $([\alpha1(I)]_3)$, 300 nm rod-shaped triple helical collagen molecules linearly aligned and cylindrically grouped as fibrils. Parallel fibrils gathered into fibres 10% non-collagenous proteins (phosphorylated phosphoproteins (MW 140 kDa), Gla-proteins, macromolecular proteoglycans, plasma proteins, acidic glycoproteins), water	*Tubules* (EDJ to pulp chamber); approximately 19–45,000 per mm²; coronal sigmoid curvature; 1–5 μm diameter; anastomosing branches evident (0.5 μm to 25 nm diameter); odontoblasts and processes

MW, molecular weight; kDa – kilodaltons; EDJ, enamel–dentine junction.

Table 7.2 Clinical properties that each of the dental hard tissues confers on a tooth, and those properties that an ideal restorative material should mimic

	Enamel	**Enamel–dentine junction**	**Dentine**
Clinical properties	Rigidity/brittle High compressive strength Wear resistance Translucency Dry	Scalloped Optical tint Limits crack propagation/ catastrophic failure Approximately 50 MPa bond strength	Bulk Slight elasticity/flexibility Shade Dynamic hydration: wetter, closer to the pulp (affects bonding ability)
Restorative replacement material	Dental resin composite	Dentine bonding agent Dynamic chemical bond	Glass ionomer cement

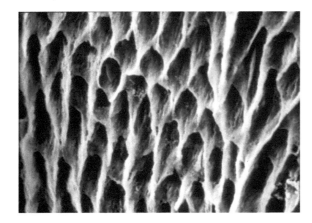

Figure 7.4 The tooth's view of an acid etch-retained resin bond. The enamel was etched, washed, bonded, and then dissolved away using a strong acid. The acid-resistant resin layer was retained. It can be seen to have flowed into the prism boundary regions (field width 80 μm). (Courtesy of Professor A Boyde.)

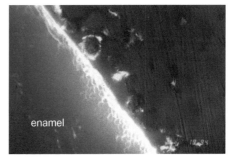

enamel

Figure 7.5 The interface between etched and bonded enamel prisms and a restoration. The bonding agent has been labelled with a yellow fluorescent dye (fluorescein), and its penetration around the horseshoe-shaped enamel prisms can be seen. Enamel prisms are easily separated from one another in the lateral walls of a cavity such as this, especially if the restoration shrinks (field width 500 μm).

2. After washing the acid etch gel off and drying the enamel thoroughly, a layer of fluid unfilled hydrophobic bonding resin (i.e. the resin without filler particles) is placed on to the etched enamel surface. This resin can flow easily into the micro-undercuts created by the etching process, and it is then light cured. Note that the chemistry of the unfilled fluid bonding resin is not the same as that of a dentine bonding agent (see later).

3. The final composite can then be placed on the layer of photo-cured bonding resin, in small angled increments (to lessen the effects of polymerization shrinkage), and photo-cured to form the final contoured restoration (see Figure 7.5).

When bonding to enamel, consideration must be given to the quality of the prismatic structure, as this is critical to adhesion. Unprepared young enamel may still retain a layer of *aprismatic* enamel—that is, the final layers of enamel to be laid down before completion of enamel

development. This layer is void of enamel prisms as the elongated Tomes' processes of the enamel-producing cells, the ameloblasts, had already retracted as enamel deposition was nearing completion. Up to 10 microns in thickness, this layer is often removed in normal function due to the normal causes of tooth surface loss (erosion, abrasion, and attrition; see Chapter 1, Section 1.3). Prisms that have been sectioned/cracked/pulled apart during tooth preparation with rotary instrumentation, and whose bases do not reach the enamel–dentine junction (EDJ) intact, are described as being *unsupported*. These prisms are inherently weak, and if bonded to they will pull apart physically under the stresses exerted on them by the curing resin composite. This will lead to relatively short-term marginal failure within the enamel (i.e. cohesive enamel failure). In theory, if supported prisms are cut at, or close to, 90° to their long axis (i.e. clinically, the enamel margin is lightly bevelled) then the deleterious effects of shrinkage stress at the margins may be reduced, as prisms possess greater tensile and compressive strength along their c-axes, as opposed to perpendicular to the c-axes. Enamel that has lost much of the underlying dentine beneath it (*undermined* enamel) will need to have this replaced with a suitable material prior to the resin composite–enamel bond being created.

Resin composite and dentine: dentine bonding agents

The fundamental clinical problem is to achieve intimate compatibility of two immiscible substrates—dentine is hydrophilic (likes water and is innately wet), whereas methacrylate resins are hydrophobic (water-hating). Therefore a *dentine bonding agent (DBA)* is required as an adhesive between the two. DBAs have three generic components:

- *Etch*: the first stage of the process, which has the following effects on dentine:
  - It removes the dentine smear layer created by the cavity preparation process (see Figure 7.6).
  - It helps to unblock and widen the dentine tubule orifices.
  - It demineralizes the dentine surface, thereby exposing the network of collagen in the dentine matrix (see Table 7.1).

- *Primer*: a bifunctional coupling molecule (e.g. hydrophilic HEMA—hydroxyethylmethacrylate) which has one functional group that likes water, so is compatible with the moist collagen in dentine,

and another that likes resin, so is compatible with the bond/composite. The primer is carried into the moist collagen fibrillar network using a solvent (water, acetone, or alcohol), displacing the water molecules from the collagen and permitting the primer to enter the micro- and nano-spaces created around the collagen fibrils after the etching process. Other monomers that have been shown to promote successful bonding to hydroxyapatite and calcium ions include the MDP monomer (10-methacryloyloxydecyl dihydrogen phosphate). This has a terminal double bond group for polymerization, a hydrophobic alkylene group to maintain the balance between hydrophobic and hydrophilic properties, and a hydrophilic phosphate group for acid demineralization and chemical bonding to tooth structure.

- *Bond*: this can be considered simply as the resin component of the composite without the filler particles. A mixture of low-viscosity monomers able to penetrate the spaces not occupied by the primer monomers, it can be cured in the conventional way and then finally the resin composite placed incrementally (chemically cross-linking to the monomers in the air-inhibited layer of the bond) and the restoration completed.

Each of these sensitive stages needs to be accomplished in optimal clinical conditions to enable a successful bond to be created between resin composite and dentine. The status of the collagen network on the cut dentine surface is of prime importance—it is the penetration of the primer and bond into these micro-/nano-spaces that provides the integrity of the seal and bond between resin composite and dentine. This zone of collagen penetration is known as the *hybrid zone*, and it can be 0.5–15 µm thick. Note that the thickness of the hybrid zone is less important than its continuity and integrity along the bonding interface. Any significant gaps in the hybrid zone will reduce the quality of the seal and ultimately of the bond. Penetration of the bonding agent into the dentine tubules will also play a part in reinforcing the bond strength (see Figure 7.7). DBAs can also be used on enamel instead of the unfilled bonding resin described earlier, to simplify the overall bonding process, but note that the chemistries of unfilled bonding resin (for enamel only) and DBAs (for both dentine and enamel) are different. There are numerous clinical presentations of DBAs from different manufacturers, and a simple classification system dependent on the three stages described previously is presented in Table 7.3. In Chapter 8, Table 8.12 outlines in more detail the differences in the clinical techniques employed for each type of system.

7.2.4 Classification of dentine bonding agents

Type 1 (three-bottle or three-step bonding systems)

Each of the three clinical steps is completed separately. Ideally, dentine should be etched for 10–15 seconds and enamel for 20 seconds using 37% orthophosphoric acid, which is then washed away thoroughly (for 10 seconds) and dried until the enamel appears frosty white. The primer contains water, so the over-dried exposed collagen on the dentine surface will rehydrate up to a point, thus permitting the primer and bond to penetrate the collagen network. However, over-etching coupled with incomplete rehydration of the collagen might leave unfilled

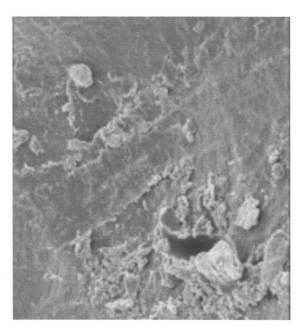

Figure 7.6 Dentine smear layer (a tenacious layer of organic and inorganic cutting debris usually < 20 µm thick) imaged using scanning electron microscopy: this can be a barrier to good bonding, and is normally removed or modified using acids (field width 500 µm).

Q7.2: A dentine smear layer is illustrated in Figure 7.6. How is the smear layer created?

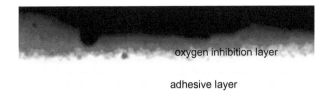

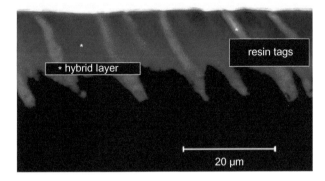

Figure 7.7 A fluorescent micrograph of a dentine bonding agent, showing penetration of the red-labelled (rhodamine) primer into the collagen network and tubules in dentine, forming the hybrid zone up to 15 μm thick (nano-retention) as well as resin tags (micro-retention). The yellow-labelled (fluorescein) adhesive uses its oxygen-inhibition layer to aid adherence to the composite. (Courtesy of S. Sauro.)

micro-/nano-porosities within the depth of the hybrid zone, and subsequent fluid movement might lead to post-operative sensitivity and bond degradation over time. Even though the clinical technique sensitivity is greater for these type 1 systems, due to the three separate steps, it is universally accepted that type 1, three-bottle systems provide a good-quality and reliable bond, and they have been used for many years as the gold standard for dentine bond measurement in laboratory studies.

Type 2 (two-bottle or two-stage, 'total etch' or 'etch and rinse' adhesives)

The clinical stages have been simplified into two steps—an initial etch, which is then rinsed away thereby removing the smear layer. In type 2 systems it is imperative not to over-dry the exposed collagen network, as this cannot be rehydrated by the contents of the second bottle containing both the primer and the bond (see Figure 7.8). A technique of 'moist bonding' must be employed after washing off the etchant gel, wicking the 'puddles' of excess water away using cotton wool pledgets, paper points, or very gentle air drying (see Chapter 8). This will ensure that the collagen network remains erect and supported, so more conducive to bond penetration (see Figure 7.9). The primer and bond are combined, and it is essential to evaporate the solvent carrier (acetone or alcohol based), as any remnants will contaminate and weaken the final bond. This procedure also thins the adhesive on the cavity walls, and the operator must ensure that there is enough adhesive present before the photo-curing stage (the cavity walls must appear shiny). Therefore multiple applications of the adhesive (primer and bond together) may be required prior to placing the resin composite restoration.

Type 3 (weaker self-etching primers)

The acid phosphate monomers in the primer act as the etchant, so no separate etching/rinsing/drying phase or moist bonding technique is required. The dentine is etched sufficiently to partially dissolve the smear layer and expose the collagen network. However, uncut

Table 7.3 A classification system for modern dentine bonding agents indicating the effect on the smear layer, and presentation options of the three stages—etch, primer, and bond—with some UK market examples

Type	Smear	Etch	Prime	Bond	Examples
1 three bottle (4th generation)	Remove				Adper Scotchbond MP Optibond FL
2 etch & rinse (5th generation)	Remove				Optibond Solo Prime & Bond NT/XP One Step Plus Scothbond Universal
3 mild self-etch (6th generation)	Dissolve				Clearfil SE Bond/Protect Bond
4 strong self-etch (7th generation)	Dissolve				Scotchbond Universal Xeno III; I Bond One up bond F Plus
		Milder self-etching primer			Fuji Bond LC; G Bond; Tri S Bond

A box that extends across two columns represents different components of dental adhesives being blended together.

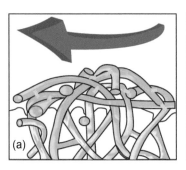 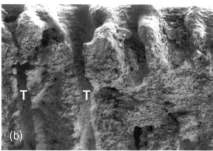 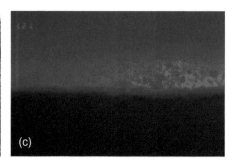

Figure 7.8 **(a)** Diagram showing collagen fibres in dentine that have been over-dried after etching. They have collapsed, so neither the primer nor bond can penetrate into the nano-spaces within the collagen network (red arrow). **(b)** A scanning electron micrograph (field width 75 μm) showing an over-dried cut dentine surface with a collapsed collagen network (T, dentine tubule cut longitudinally). **(c)** Fluorescent confocal microscopic image (field width 250 μm) showing the bonding agent labelled with rhodamine (red upper portion). The resin composite can be seen in the top half of the image and the very faint outlines of dentinal tubules in the lower half. Note that as the dentine has been over-dried (see Figure 7.8a), there has been no penetration of the collagen network or tubules, and the resulting bond and seal will be poor. (Figure 7.8 (a) courtesy of D. Ziskind.)

Q7.3: What are the dark irregular shapes outlined within the rhodamine-labelled (red) upper portion in Figure 7.8 (c)?

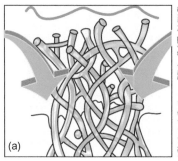 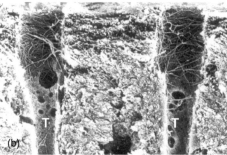 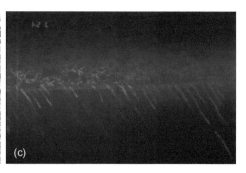

Figure 7.9 **(a)** Diagram showing collagen fibres in dentine that have been kept moist, so the network is upright with micro-/nano-spaces available to accept the primer and bond (green arrows). **(b)** An environmental scanning electron micrograph (field width 75 μm) showing moist collagen on the cut dentine surface. Individual collagen fibrils can be easily detected, and the orifices of two tubules have been clearly widened by the etching process (T, dentine tubule cut longitudinally). **(c)** Fluorescent confocal microscopic image (field width 250 μm) showing the bonding agent labelled with a red dye penetrating the moist collagen network on the dentine surface (nano-mechanical retention) and into the tubules (micro-mechanical retention). Note the thin red diffuse band at the interface between dentine and composite (arrow); this is the *hybrid zone* (10 μm thick). (Figure 7.9 (a) courtesy of D. Ziskind. Figure 7.9 (b) courtesy of Bart van Meerbeek.)

enamel margins may be etched less efficiently, leading to a distinct possibility of stained margins of restorations in the long term (see Figure 7.10).

This problem may be prevented by pre-etching the enamel margins with 37% orthophosphoric acid for 20 seconds, converting the whole clinical process to one similar to a type 1, three-stage system (see Chapter 8). The solvent again must be evaporated after the acidic primer is rubbed on to the dentine surface as in the type 2 systems.

Type 4 (stronger self-etching all-in-one systems)

Clinically, these are the simplest to use as there is a single application step, but the three bonding stages (etch, prime, and bond) are somewhat compromised. These are the most recent additions to the market, and laboratory studies on sound enamel and dentine show not only favourable bond strengths but also the presence of water blisters in the adhesive layer as it acts as a semi-permeable membrane, drawing water from the wet dentine tubules. As hydrolysis of polymeric dentine bonds occurs, there is evidence that marginal discoloration is more of an

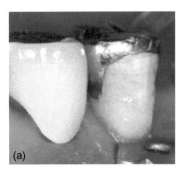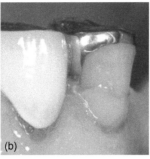

(a)   (b)

Figure 7.10 (a) Resin composite class V buccal cervical restoration LL5 placed using a type 3 self-etching primer dentine bonding agent. **(b)** The same restoration, 10 years later.

Q7.4: Look at Figure 7.10 (a) and (b). Can you spot the difference between the two and explain the reason for the difference?

issue with these adhesives. However, vigorous evaporation of the water-based solvent in the adhesive may reduce this problem.

7.2.5 Clinical issues with dentine bonding agents

- *Technique sensitivity*: The steps involved in dentine bonding require high levels of moisture control intra-orally, and appropriate handling of the dental materials themselves. For example, if volatile solvents are allowed to evaporate naturally from bottles of adhesive when the lids are not replaced after dispensing, the chemistry is irreversibly adversely affected, so bonding will be impaired. Primers and bond need to be agitated well into the tooth surface, and all these steps must be followed to obtain a successful bond. Avoid the temptation to take clinical short cuts and omit stages of the bonding procedure!

- *Packaging instructions*: Familiarization with the steps in the bonding process is essential, and teamwork with the nurse is vital in order to place the various materials in the correct order, with speed and precision. Single-dose capsules/foils/bubble-packs can be of assistance, reducing wastage and improving infection control procedures.

- *Shelf-life*: If kept refrigerated, the shelf-life of most DBAs is good. Volatile solvents need to be kept tightly stoppered, and as the materials are light sensitive, the use of blacked-out bottles is advised.

- *Suitable substrate*: Most studies on DBAs use sound enamel and dentine as the tooth surface to which to bond, often on extracted teeth. The histological properties of teeth *in vivo* may be quite different, and also the quality of the hard tissues will vary depending on the amount of carious tooth structure that has been retained. Therefore a comprehensive understanding is required of the state of the collagen network and mineral prior to using the DBA. More recent publications have used caries-affected dentine substrates *in vitro* and show clinically acceptable bond strengths (15–28 MPa).

- *Hydrolysis*: This is the major factor in the long-term degradation of the bond interface. The residual monomers will be affected by the water transition through vital dentine, thus ultimately compromising

the seal and bond. Therefore a good-quality peripheral enamel seal is essential for the long-term success of adhesive bonding. Matrix metalloproteinases (MMPs) released from the exposed collagen (see Chapter 1), and activated in the caries acidic environment, may account for the failure of the adhesive bond in both caries-affected and sound dentine by accelerating collagen fibril cleavage. This in turn will cause a breakdown of the hybrid zone, thus jeopardizing the long-term adhesive seal and bond.

- *Sensitization*: These chemicals are designed to penetrate living tissue, and latex or nitrile gloves do not offer protection from resin-based materials. Therefore the dentist and nurse need to follow a 'no-touch' regimen when handling these materials.

7.2.6 Developments

The world of dental materials is constantly changing, and by the time this book is published new materials will be available for use clinically. Some of the challenges and developments are discussed in this section.

Reducing shrinkage stress and strain

Manufacturers can alleviate the problem of significant volumetric shrinkage (often leading to increased marginal stress and/or material strain) by producing low-shrink materials, or materials that impart little strain on the tooth. Such a system is illustrated by siloxane-oxirane (silorane) chemistry, as opposed to conventional methacrylates. In this system, the monomers, instead of being linear, are ring-opening and therefore, during the cationic polymerization process, less shrinkage occurs (0.9%). This chemistry requires a separate bonding agent, which is very hydrophobic, thereby minimizing the water transition through the adhesive. Another system is a dimer-acid nano-hybrid composite (based on dimer dicarbamate dimethacrylates), which exhibits polymerization-induced phase separation (expansion) on curing, thereby reducing some of the effects of polymerization shrinkage. Although these low-shrink materials have been shown to be effective, dentists are still using conventional resin composites, perhaps indicating that the problems of shrinkage stress can be mitigated by careful handling. Conversely, the 'bulk-fill' material developments (see Section 7.2.2) indicate that low stress/low viscosity composites that simplify restoration placement can become popular—time will tell if these are successful clinically.

Dentine bonding agents

With the advent of low-shrink composites, the importance of direct bond strengths may lessen and more emphasis may be placed on the ionic interaction between the materials and tooth structure. Medicinal ions could be transferred from the adhesive to help to remineralize the enamel or dentine, or act as anti-bacterial agents.

'Self-adhesive composite'

The ultimate development, a simple to use, self-adhesive composite restorative material, has been marketed, but bond strengths to dental hard tissues are not yet good enough for it to be recommended for regular use. The technology will not be long in the offing, however, as clinically successful self-etch resin cements do exist, currently used to adhere indirect restorations and root canal posts to teeth.

7.3 Glass ionomer cement

Glass ionomer cement (GIC) is a water-based, plastic direct dental restorative cement formed from an acid–base reaction between a poly-alkenoic acid and ion-leachable fluoro-calcium (strontium) aluminosilicate glass particles.

7.3.1 History

GIC was developed as a biocompatible, chemically adhesive plastic restorative material by Wilson and Kent in the UK in 1972.

7.3.2 Chemistry

- *Powder*: calcium fluoro-aluminosilicate glass particles with strontium (to increase radio-opacity). The silica (SiO_2—affects transparency), alumina (Al_2O_3—affects opacity and setting time, and can increase the compressive strength of the set cement), and calcium fluoride (CaF_2—the fluoride ions reduce the fusion temperature, increase the strength of the set cement, enhance translucency, and have a therapeutic effect) are the important components. These are structured ionically as a tetrahedral complex with a centrally located aluminium ion and closely localized alkaline earth cations (sodium, potassium, calcium, and strontium) to maintain electro-neutrality.

- *Liquid-polyacid*: itaconic acid copolymer solution in water plus tartaric acid (5–15%, maintains working time and assists setting reaction). Anhydrous forms have vacuum-dried polyacrylic acid incorporated into the powder and are mixed with water ± dilute solution of tartaric acid.

- *Setting reaction*: acid–base reaction with three stages:

1. *Dissolution*: sol formation from the outer layers of the glass particles as they are attacked by the polyacid, and calcium, strontium, aluminium, and fluoride ions are released.

2. *Gelation and hardening*: primarily calcium ions bind to carboxylate groups (4 to 5 minutes) producing a clinically hard surface (initial set), and a silaceous hydrogel is formed, maturing over 24 hours, with further cross-linking with aluminium ions, up to 7 days. This process causes volumetric shrinkage of up to 3%. Surface protection at this stage is advisable to ensure regulation of the movement of water molecules in and out of the hydrogel, so permitting maturation to occur.

3. *Hydration*: associated with Stage 2, this continues over 4 to 6 months, so improving the physical properties of the material. The uptake of water leads to expansion, thereby reducing the ill effects of the initial shrinkage.

7.3.3 The tooth–GIC interface

GICs have the ability to adhere chemically to mineralized dental tissues. They do this by the dynamic processes of diffusion and adsorption.

Enamel

GIC polyacid displaces phosphate and divalent Ca^{2+} ions from the hydroxyapatite, and these ions become incorporated into the GIC matrix, which sets. Subsequently the pH rises and re-precipitation of minerals at the GIC–tooth interface occurs, forming an ion-enriched layer, which is so firmly bound that when GIC restorations fail, this can be cohesive within the GIC material itself (see Figure 7.11). If the enamel

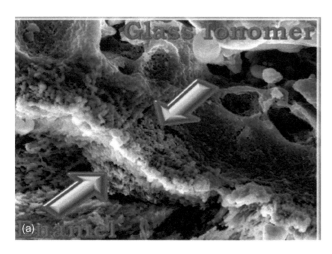
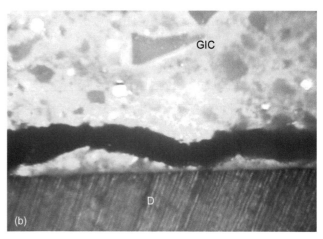

Figure 7.11 **(a)** Scanning electron microscopy image showing the interface between glass ionomer and enamel. The section surface has been etched lightly and a raised area (between the arrows) shows the *ion-enriched* layer at the tooth–restoration interface (field width 10 μm). **(b)** Fractured GIC–tooth interface (D) showing the cohesive failure common to these materials. The *ion-enriched* layer is still attached to the tooth (field width 300 μm). (Figure 7.11 (a) courtesy of Professor Hien Ngo.)

Q7.5: What is responsible for the cohesive fracture in Figure 7.11 (b)?

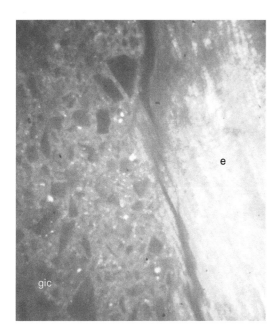

Figure 7.12 Photomicrograph of glass ionomer cement having pulled apart enamel prisms and caused cohesive failure in the enamel (e; black arrow) (field width 100 μm).

Q7.6: What are the irregular-shaped particles within the GIC in Figure 7.12?

prisms have been damaged/fractured/pulled apart in creating the cavity, the mineralized component of the interface can also fail cohesively due to the initial shrinkage stresses generated by the setting GIC (see Figure 7.12).

Dentine–collagen

Adhesion to collagen may occur through hydrogen bond formation or metallic ion bridging between carboxyl groups of the polyacid and collagen.

Dentine–tubules

There is limited evidence to argue for any significant micro-mechanical retention by the penetration of dentine tubules. The penetration is slight (< 5 μm), and the tensile strength of GIC in this proportion is poor, so is unlikely to contribute to retention.

Conditioning

Conditioning is the process by which both enamel and dentine are 'freshened' or pre-activated prior to the placement of freshly mixed GIC. The acid used is 10% polyacrylic acid for 10 seconds, which is then washed off and the surface dried gently, in order to:

- remove/modify the smear layer and expose calcium and phosphate ions on the mineralized surface
- increase the surface energy of the tooth surface to allow improved wettability of the GIC as it is placed on the tooth surface.

Dentine conditioner is mildly acidic, so it neither demineralizes the dentine excessively, nor opens up dentine tubules. Note that this conditioning step is not the same as the 'conditioners' used in resin composite retention—that material, even though sharing the same nomenclature (especially in the USA), is a much stronger acid etch (37% orthophosphoric acid).

7.3.4 Clinical uses of GIC relating to its properties

GICs are used conventionally as:

- luting cements for indirect restorations, where the powder:liquid ratio is closer to 1.5:1 (lower viscosity to improve cavity margin adaptation)
- direct restorative material, with a powder:liquid ratio of > 3:1 (stiffer, high-viscosity material)
- indirect pulp protection, with a powder:liquid ratio of 1.5:1, covering a direct pulp capping agent (e.g. calcium hydroxide or MTA) or in the depths of a cavity with very close proximity to the pulp, beneath an amalgam restoration (see Chapter 5, Section 5.11).

As a restorative material, the best physical properties (tensile and compressive strengths) of GIC are exhibited when the high-viscosity material is used in thick section, but GICs are still not universally recommended for *long-term* stress-bearing restorations (e.g. posterior occlusal restorations). Internal cavity line angles should be smooth and rounded prior to placement.

- *Fracture resistance*: original GICs were brittle and prone to fracture under heavy occlusal loading. Modern higher-viscosity derivatives have improved fracture toughness, but there is still little clinical evidence and justification for them being used routinely as *long-term* restorations in the posterior load-bearing dentition.
- *Abrasion resistance*: again generally poor, but modern resin-based surface coating systems (e.g. G-Coat Plus, GC Japan) can help to regulate the long-term water uptake and provide a protective and aesthetic coating, so improving this quality.
- *Physical properties*: compressive shear strengths, thermal expansion, and diffusivity have all improved with developments in GIC science. Modern materials appear to have some properties approaching more closely those of natural dentine.
- *Fluoride release*: fluoride ions are released initially at high levels, which fall away 8–10 weeks after placement. The fluoride ions are captured within the siliceous hydrogel matrix and can pass in and out of this to the tooth surface, so prompting the description that it can act as a 'fluoride reservoir', recharging from the high doses of professional fluoride application. There is contrary evidence, however, which argues that the fluoride release effect is of subclinical value after initial placement.
- *Aesthetics*: improvements have been made with better shade and translucency of modern GICs. Water uptake and high solubility affect the long-term stability of colour and translucency in restorations, but coating the surface just after placement or veneering the surface with composite at a later date are potential solutions.

7.3.5 Developments

As with dental resin composites, GIC material science is continuously evolving. Developments include the following:

- the speed, control, and conversion rate of the initial set, with fast-setting materials on the market taking 90 seconds to reach a carvable stage

- improving the physical properties in order to enable more reliable use in posterior, load-bearing cavities with the potential use of ceramic nano-filler technology or developing the use of N-vinyl pyrollidone-containing polyacids (NVPs) in the matrix polymer

- improving the wear resistance, polishability, and aesthetics of the final restoration with advances in resin-based coating systems, applied after finishing the restoration

- greater use of the ionic-exchange potential to introduce other ions to help to remineralize, repair tooth structure, and confer antibacterial effects.

7.4 Resin-modified glass ionomer cement (RM-GIC) and poly-acid modified resin composite ('compomer')

The description of these materials as 'light-cured GICs' should be avoided.

7.4.1 Chemistry

RM-GICs

RM-GICs essentially have the same chemistry as a conventional GIC with the addition of the hydrophilic resin, HEMA (hydroxyethyl-methacrylate), bis-GMA, and other photo-initiators. They set with a combination reaction: acid–base between the glass particles and polyalkenoic acid (as previously described) and also light-cured polymerization reaction of the resin (similar to that of a resin composite). The resin in RM-GICs can also undergo chemical polymerization due to an intrinsic redox (reduction–oxidation) reaction, so auto-curing over time (approximately 1 month) into a fully set material. Due to the fact that the HEMA resin is hydrophilic, there is a risk that after the initial snap-setting process, water is absorbed which might lead to medium- to long-term degradation and colour instability when used as the definitive restorative material (see Figure 7.13). These materials at a low powder:liquid ratio form the basis of widely used luting systems in fixed prosthodontics. Clinical examples include Fuji II LC®, Vitremer®, and Ketac Nano®.

Poly-acid modified composites

These are materials that are primarily resin-based, with some GIC chemistry incorporated, but not enough to promote an acid–base setting reaction. They essentially require light activation to promote the polymerization chain reaction. They cannot adhere chemically to tooth structure as do conventional GICs, as the acid–base reaction only occurs over a prolonged time period, after the initial set of the resin component. Therefore dentine bonding agents are a prerequisite for retention of these materials within a cavity. The original example of this class of material is Dyract®.

7.4.2 Clinical indications

Both of these materials can be used as provisional or definitive shade-matched tooth-coloured adhesive restoratives. However, there is some evidence that the colour stability of RM-GICs might be suspect over longer periods, due to the extent of water absorption that occurs (see Figure 7.13).

RM-GICs may also be used as a base in an adhesive *layered/laminate/'sandwich'* restoration with an overlying composite completely covering the RM-GIC base (a closed restoration). However, there is clinical evidence that these types of restoration are more prone to long-term failure, especially at the interfaces between the different materials. It is the authors' opinion that the *layered/laminate/'sandwich'* restoration should be limited to the placement of a resin composite veneer over the exposed occlusal surface of large GICs/RM-GICs at least 6 months after the GIC restoration has been placed to allow for its full maturation, so maximizing its physical and chemical properties.

When indirect chair-side or laboratory-made restorations are used, some form of cementation (or luting) is required (see Section 7.7.3), and the use of self-etching low-viscosity derivatives of the RMGIC technology has become popular for such an application. Although the adhesive bond strengths of these materials may be inferior to those of a multi-stage light- and self-cured resin adhesive system, used in conjunction with low-viscosity dual-cured composite luting cement their handling simplicity will produce more reliable everyday clinical performance. An example of this type of material is RelyX Unicem® (3MESPE).

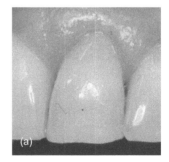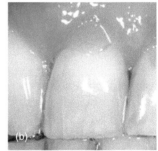

Figure 7.13 (a) RM-GIC buccal cervical Class V restoration UL1 with good aesthetic properties initially. **(b)** The same restoration 7 years later, showing obvious intrinsic discoloration due to water absorption.

7.5 Dental amalgam

Dental amalgam (one of the oldest direct plastic restorative materials still in use) is an alloy of one or more metals including silver (Ag), tin (Sn), zinc (Zn), copper (Cu), and tiny amounts of some minor elements (palladium, platinum, indium) with mercury (Hg). Its use is rapidly on the decline worldwide as:

- Patients demand more aesthetic restorations and can appreciate the benefits of simple tooth-preserving restore/repair cycles of minimally invasive treatment.

- Health and safety and environmental concerns are raised about the use and disposal of mercury. This can be mitigated against by the use of appropriate traps in surgery waste water systems (compulsory in the UK). The United Nations Environment Programme (UNEP) 2013 Minamata Convention on Mercury has declared that the use of dental amalgam will be phased down, as caries prevention strategies and research into alternative restorative materials develop.

- Adhesive materials have developed with significantly improved bonding capabilities to sound and caries-affected tooth structure.

- Principles of minimally invasive operative dentistry have been embraced, producing smaller, less mechanically retentive cavities to restore, so promoting the use of adhesive materials.

- Caries control/management strategies have evolved with a better understanding of the histopathology of the disease.

7.5.1 Chemistry

- Silver (75–70%), tin (27–29%), copper (< 7% low Cu, > 12% high Cu), and trace metallic elements (< 1%) are presented as phases—γ gamma (Ag_3Sn), ε epsilon (Cu_3Sn), and d dispersant (Ag-Cu eutectic alloy)—and mixed with mercury (triturated in an amalgamator unit) to form an alloy (amalgamation reaction), so producing the intrinsic strength and mechanical properties of the set material.

- Metal phases are presented as ingots which are then made into lathe-cut particles. Alternatively, molten alloy is sprayed into an inert atmosphere and atomized into spherical particles. The final powder may be an admix of the two particle types. The particle size and shape have an effect on the ease of packing of the triturated amalgam into a cavity; spherical particle alloys require less force to condense into a cavity, resulting in fewer voids.

- Copper: modern alloys are high Cu alloys with > 12% Cu (single composition or dispersion-modified Cu-enriched alloys). The inclusion of copper improves corrosion and creep resistance and strengthens the set material by reducing unwanted Sn-Hg γ_2 (gamma 2) phase in the set amalgam.

- Zinc: > 0.01% Zn was introduced to scavenge oxygen when casting the metal ingots. The use of an inert atmosphere during the manufacture of spherical particles now makes the inclusion of zinc redundant. Inclusion of zinc led to increased hygroscopic expansion due to water contamination during placement, but may increase marginal strength.

7.5.2 Physical properties

- *Strength*: high compressive and tensile strengths several days after placement. Care is required when checking the occlusion immediately after condensation and carving, as the amalgam may be brittle at this stage. High Cu alloys have a greater strength and are used in large load-bearing posterior restorations. Amalgam is weak in thin section and requires at least 2 mm thickness to support itself. Therefore cavity design is important for this reason as well as for mechanical retention via undercuts and for support.

- *Corrosion*: an electrochemical breakdown due to the interaction between any metal and its surroundings. Low Cu amalgams corroded quickly and extensively, so sealing the micro-gaps between the cavity wall and restoration. High Cu alloys are more resistant to corrosion and corrosion fatigue at the margins. Amalgam surfaces can oxidize over time, leading to surface corrosion or even breakdown, resulting in pitting and surface deficiencies.

- *Rigidity:* the modulus of elasticity of amalgam is high but not as rigid as enamel.

- *Dimensional changes:* after minor setting contraction, water uptake during setting (especially in low Cu, Zn-containing alloys) can lead to hydrogen production and expansion, resulting in pain. Thermal expansion can also occur to a degree further than normal tooth structure, so fine surface polishing, the friction of which will generate heat, should be undertaken with due care.

7.5.3 Bonded and sealed amalgams

Amalgam restorations obtain retention within a cavity macro-mechanically, achieved by making undercut preparations (where the base of the cavity is wider than its opening) or using slots/grooves, root canal posts, or the pulp chamber and root canal orifices themselves (Nayyar core; see Figure 7.14). All of these require excessive amounts of tooth structure to be removed or damaged to some extent, thus ultimately weakening the remaining tissue—not particularly minimally invasive! Dentine pins have been used to retain amalgam in larger cavities where cusps are missing. There is clear evidence that correct placement of dentine pins tends to significantly increase the stresses in an already weakened tooth, leading to ultimate catastrophic failure of the restoration and tooth. It is the authors' opinion that dentine pins should not be used in modern dentistry, as alternative methods and materials now exist, including self-curing adhesive luting cements to couple the cavity walls to the amalgam restoration.

Bonded amalgams

An adhesive, chemically cured, resin-based luting cement is used to seal the exposed dentine tubules after cavity preparation, bonding to the dentine mineral and collagen (as with resin composites) and micromechanically interlocking simultaneously with the freshly condensed amalgam as they both set (see Chapter 8, Section 8.9). Chemical bonds with metal oxides forming in the set amalgam may form, but these have

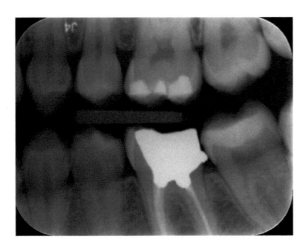

Figure 7.14 Left bitewing radiograph showing an amalgam Nayyar core LL7. Note how the 'amalgam pins' extend into the coronal aspects of the endodontically treated root canals, to aid retention after the gutta-percha was removed. The bulk of amalgam will also confer strength on the restoration. For the clinical steps to place a Nayyar core, see Chapter 8.

Q7.7: What problem can you see with the restoration in Figure 7.14 and how can it be treated? What do you think should be considered as part of the long-term management of this tooth?

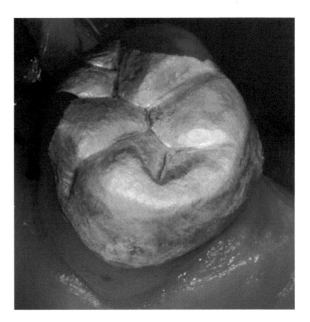

Figure 7.15 Broken down mandibular molar restored with a large load-bearing amalgam restoration. (Courtesy L. Mackenzie.)

Q7.8: At what stage of restoration placement has the photograph in Figure 7.15 been taken, and what stage is left to complete?

little clinical significance for retention in the long term. The evidence for their routine use is inconclusive, but the procedure might be beneficial when repairing old fractured large amalgams with new amalgam.

Sealed amalgams

As modern high copper alloys corrode less and so do not adequately seal the spaces at the tooth–amalgam interface, a flowable resin/dentine bonding agent can be used to coat the surface of the tooth–amalgam interface after condensation, carving, and finishing. This can penetrate the micro-gaps at the marginal interface which form during the setting process, so reducing the likelihood of marginal leakage and the risk of subsequent caries. A dentine bonding agent may also be used to seal the dentine cavity walls prior to placement of the amalgam restoration.

7.5.4 Modern indications for the use of amalgam

In the current climate of more acceptable tooth-coloured alternatives and minimally invasive dentistry, as well as the ever growing environmental concerns about the safety and disposal of mercury, the use of dental amalgam is becoming more limited. Due to the presence of alternatives, the uses of amalgam may reasonably be restricted to large posterior load-bearing restorations or as a core material for crowns (see Figure 7.15 and Chapter 8).

7.6 Temporary (intermediate) and provisional restorative materials

7.6.1 Characteristics

Temporary restorative materials should ideally be:

- simple for both dentist and nurse to handle clinically
- easy to remove to allow final placement of the definitive restoration
- materials that do not interfere with the setting/bonding chemistry of any definitive restorative material
- durable enough to last in the oral cavity for several weeks

- cheap and biocompatible.

Provisional restorative materials should have all of the characteristics described in the previous list, and ideally they should be:

- durable enough to last in the oral cavity for several months
- as aesthetic as possible.

The boundary between a provisional and definitive restorative material is nowadays quite blurred, as many adhesive restorative materials combine both functions.

7.6.2 Chemistry

- Radio-opaque, polymer-reinforced zinc oxide:eugenol cements (e.g. Kalzinol®, Sedanol®, pre-mixed Intermediate Restorative Material, or IRM®). Quick setting and easy to spatulate and load into cavities, but must not be used where resin composites will follow, as the eugenol affects the polymerization chain reaction adversely.

- Glass ionomer cements (see previous sections).
- Zinc polycarboxylate cements (Poly F® Plus): water-soluble, low-molecular-weight polymers of acrylic or methacrylic acid that form solid, insoluble products when mixed with specially prepared zinc oxide powder. The resulting cement adheres to dental enamel and can also be used as a luting agent.

7.7 Calcium silicate-based cements

7.7.1 History

Calcium silicate-based cements were first introduced to operative dentistry in 1993, when Torabinejad developed a formula based on ordinary Portland cement (OPC), which was intended primarily for use as an endodontic material (e.g. in root end/perforation repairs). A mineral trioxide aggregate (MTA), which is composed principally of tri-calcium silicate, di-calcium silicate, tri-calcium aluminate, and tetra-calcium aluminoferrite, its operative dental applications were somewhat limited due to the protracted working and setting time of several hours.

In 2010, Biodentine™ (Septodont, France), a quicker setting calcium silicate-based restorative cement, was introduced to the market. This cement was developed as a dentine replacement material, a novel clinical application for this family of materials, with the intention that it would function as a direct coronal restoration. The comparatively short working/setting time (approximately 12 minutes) enables the use of this cement for clinical restorative procedures, which would be impossible with modern MTAs that achieve only an initial set within 3–4 hours.

7.7.2 Chemistry and interactions with the tooth

The faster-setting calcium silicate cement (Biodentine™) is composed principally of a highly purified tri-calcium silicate powder that is prepared synthetically in the laboratory *de novo*, rather than being derived from a clinker product of cement manufacture. In addition, Biodentine™ contains di-calcium silicate, calcium carbonate, and zirconium dioxide as a radio-opacifier. The powder is dispensed in a two-part capsule to which is added an aliquot of hydration liquid, composed of water, calcium chloride (to accelerate the setting reaction), and a reducing agent.

Similar to OPC, calcium silicate-based dental cements set via a hydration reaction. Although the chemical reactions taking place during the hydration are more complex, the conversion of the anhydrous phases into corresponding hydrates can be simplified as follows:

$$2Ca_3SiO_5 + 7H2O \longrightarrow 3CaO.2SiO_2.4H_2O + 3Ca(OH)_2 + energy$$
$$\textbf{C3S} + \textbf{water} \longrightarrow \textbf{CSH} + \textbf{CH}$$
$$2Ca_2SiO_4 + 5H_2O \longrightarrow 3CaO.2SiO_2.4H_2O + Ca(OH)_2 + energy$$
$$\textbf{C2S} + water \longrightarrow \textbf{CSH} + \textbf{CH}$$

This setting reaction is a dissolution–precipitation process that involves a gradual dissolution of the unhydrated calcium silicate phases (C_3S and C_2S) and the formation of hydration products, mainly calcium silicate hydrate (CSH) and calcium hydroxide (CH). The CSH precipitates as a colloidal material and grows on the surface of unhydrated calcium silicate granules, forming a matrix that binds the other components together, gradually replacing the original granules. Meanwhile, calcium hydroxide is distributed throughout the water-filled spaces present between the hydrating cement species.

The setting cement attains a high pH and this has a novel effect on the dentine. Any organic material that is exposed (e.g. demineralized collagen in caries-affected dentine) will be 'caustically etched' by the cement and then subjected to calcium ion release from the cement. This alkaline environment is very conducive to mineralization within the interface, so this material can truly be termed 'bioactive.' Equally important is the therapeutic effect on the pulp elicited by the release of calcium hydroxide, leading to reparative (tertiary) dentine formation.

7.7.3 Clinical applications

The presence of large amounts of calcium hydroxide within the set material make this material potentially useful for its therapeutic pulp effects, being more robust and resistant to dissolution compared with the traditional calcium hydroxide pulp protection materials. The fast-setting calcium silicate cement described here has sufficient compressive strength to act as a bulk replacement for dentine, but is not appropriate for long-term exposure to wear or occlusal loading in the mouth. As such, it has an appropriate use as an intermediate/provisional restorative material, especially when restoring deep carious lesions (see Figure 7.16 and Section 8.7), prior to reducing the cement height and veneering the occlusal and proximal surfaces with a material such as resin composite. The relatively slow set and maturation of this material preclude the placement of the resin composite veneer immediately on to the newly placed, initially set cement. It is better to leave it for at least 1 week to mature.

- The cut surface of the hard cement should be given a 15-second acid etch, either with phosphoric acid (followed by thorough water rinsing) or using a self-etching adhesive system, treating the cement surface much as one would dentine.

- The interface between the overlying resin composite and cement will be micro-mechanical in nature, in a similar manner to the interface between GICs and resin composites.

- The potential for the long-term acid dissolution of exposed cement under a biofilm on a proximal restoration surface would indicate that the 'closed-sandwich' type of restoration would be favoured where this is clinically achievable (see Figure 7.16).

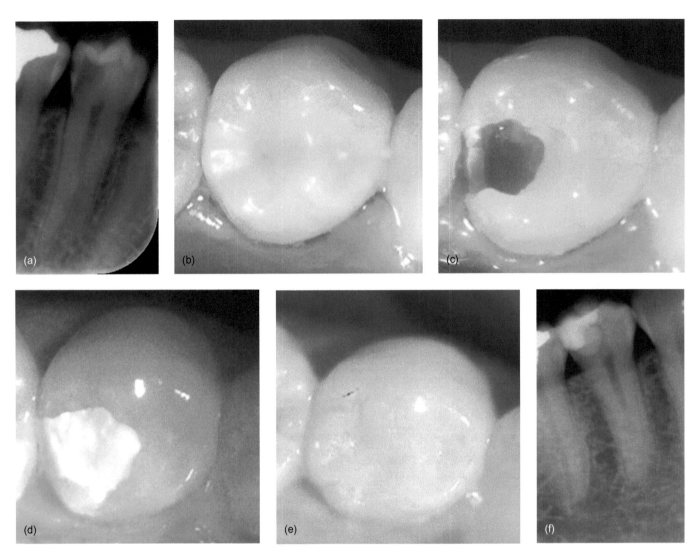

Figure 7.16 **(a)** Long cone periapical radiograph of an LR4 with a deep carious lesion distally. **(b)** The tooth was vital to the electric pulp test and exhibited the classic symptoms of an acute reversible pulpitis. A clinical decision was made to restore it minimally invasively as it was cavitated distally. **(c)** The same tooth with the lesion accessed from the occlusal aspect. Dental burs and then Carisolv™ gel were used to excavate the deepest carious dentine. No pulp exposures were created. No cavitation was observed on the mesial surface of the LR5, so this was treated non-operatively with fluoride varnish application as a preventive measure. **(d)** The Biodentine™ restoration after 1 month *in situ*. It can be seen how normal functional occlusal wear and tear has taken its toll on the restoration surface, as it is roughened significantly. **(e)** The same tooth after receiving a resin composite veneer restoration overlying the Biodentine™ beneath. This is 1 year later. **(f)** The review periapical radiograph at that time, showing no PA changes or further progression of disease. The LR4 has maintained its vitality, and the original presenting symptoms subsided fully within 1 week of the Biodentine™ being placed. Note, however, the thin radiolucent line beneath the Biodentine™ restoration in the radiograph.

Q7.8:

i   What other management regimes would you put in place to manage the patient in Figure 7.16?

ii Look at Figure 7.16 (a). What signs are evident on the radiograph that the LR4 has been resisting the caries process as it has gradually progressed through the tooth?

iii Look at Figure 7.16 (b). What are the classic symptoms of an acute reversible pulpitis? Do you think this distal lesion would be easy to detect on clinical examination?

iv Look at Figure 7.16 (c). What is Carisolv™ gel? How does it work? What quality of enamel and dentine has been retained at the base of this cavity and why?

v   Look at Figure 7.16 (f). Would you describe the resin composite veneer overlying the Biodentine™ as 'open sandwich' or 'closed sandwich'? What do you think might be the cause of the radiolucent line in the radiograph beneath the Biodentine™ restoration?

7.8 Materials and techniques for restoring the endodontically treated tooth

7.8.1 Materials

Root canal posts can be made using metals such as stainless steel, titanium, and gold, and can be directly fabricated chair-side by the dentist or indirectly cast in the laboratory. These techniques and materials have been used for many years. More recently, fibre-reinforced posts have also become popular. These posts consist of very fine glass fibres extruded in the long axis of the post and shaped within a matrix of resin, normally an epoxy or methacrylate which is then fully polymerized, but retaining a roughened surface to aid retention of the cement luting material. The shape of the post is designed to mimic the tapered anatomy of the enlarged root canal space, thus reducing the need for unnecessary root dentine removal during placement. Clinical studies have reported that direct fibre-reinforced composite posts out-perform cast and metal posts in general. However, the evidence cannot be considered conclusive.

Compared with metal posts, fibre posts (due to their flexibility and closer match to the elastic modulus of dentine) would seem to protect the root against fracture, especially when there is extensive coronal tissue breakdown/loss. The most common type of failure with fibre-reinforced composite posts is de-bonding, which normally permits re-restoration of the tooth. The current available evidence does not rule out the use of cast posts, fabricated in the dental laboratory. However, since the use of cast posts may result in a significantly greater loss of tooth structure during preparation and on failure, compared with fibre posts, their application should be limited to those cases in which no additional dentine has to be removed to allow for their cementation.

7.8.2 Root canal post cementation

Fibre and metal posts can be cemented into the root canal using all types of adhesive systems. The use of conventional two- and three-step bonding systems can be challenging, due to the difficulty in light curing the adhesive within the depths of the root canal space. Polymerization shrinkage stresses are also likely to develop in the root canal, which is a very confined space with an unfavourably high C factor (see Chapter 6, Section 6.3.1). For this reason, self-etching adhesive cements based on resin-modified glass ionomer cement technology have become very popular, as they are easy to use, create a uniform layer of cement along the root canal walls, and still allow the use of conventional two- and three-step adhesive systems to more effectively bond the resin composite core to the residual coronal tooth structure.

7.9 Suggested further reading

Darvell BW (2009) *Material Science for Dentistry*, 9 th edn. Cambridge: Woodhead Publishing Ltd. <www.woodheadpublishing.com/en/book.aspx?bookID=1547>

Curtis RV, Watson TF (eds) (2008) *Dental Biomaterials: imaging, testing and modelling*. Cambridge: Woodhead Publishing Ltd. <www.woodheadpublishing.com/en/book.aspx?bookID=1347>

7.10 Answers to self-test questions

Q7.1: What properties of the resin composite are affected by monomer chain length?

A: The viscosity of the uncured material and the degree of polymerization shrinkage (see text).

Q7.2: A dentine smear layer is illustrated in Figure 7.6. How is the smear layer created?

A: By the friction generated from any cutting instrument on the tooth surface (hand instrument or rotary). Air abrasion produces a layer similar to a smear layer created from organic/inorganic chip debris and abrasive particles.

Q7.3: What are the dark irregular shapes outlined within the rhodamine-labelled (red) upper portion in Figure 7.8 (c)?

A: These are the irregular silica-based filler particles within the resin composite.

Q7.4: Look at Figure 7.10 (a) and (b). Can you spot the difference between the two and explain the reason for the difference?

A: Note the dark discoloration on the superior margin of the restoration–enamel interface. This is due to the enamel not being as efficiently etched by the weaker self-etching primer. This has led to a less well-sealed adhesive bond, which has gradually picked up stain over the last decade of use. Pre-etching the enamel with 37% orthophosphoric acid etch can alleviate this problem.

Q7.5: What is responsible for the cohesive fracture in Figure 7.11(b)?

A: Phase 2 of the setting reaction with the formation of calcium and aluminium cross-links coupled with potential dehydration of the GIC.

Q7.6: What are the irregular-shaped particles within the GIC in Figure 7.12?

A: Unreacted fluoro-calcium aluminosilicate glass particles.

Q7.7: What problem can you see with the restoration in Figure 7.14 and how can it be treated? What do you think should be considered as part of the long-term management of this tooth?

A: Note the distal amalgam overhang, caused by inadequate adaptation of the matrix band when originally packing the cavity. This may be removed using fine burs (if clinical access is available) and interproximal amalgam finishing strips. If not, the long-term management of the tooth may involve the placement of an indirect full coverage cast restoration (e.g. a metal ceramic or full gold crown), and during the tooth preparation for this the overhang will be automatically removed.

Q7.8: At what stage of restoration placement has the photograph in Figure 7.15 been taken, and what stage is left to complete?

A: Just after the amalgam has been packed, circumferential matrix band removed, and the restoration finished. This means that the margins, contour, surface finish, contact points, and occlusion have all been checked. The next stage might be to polish the restoration to smooth the surface, thereby reducing potential plaque accumulation. However, polishing techniques must use water cooling to avoid an increase in frictional heat causing damage to the pulp (see Figure 6.1(b) in Chapter 6 for the final result).

Q7.9:

i   What other management regimes would you put in place to manage the patient in Figure 7.16?

A: A preventive regime consisting of OHI, dietary advice, and use of fluoride. Ensuring that the caries risk of this patient is brought under control, with regular review consultations to assess the patient's adherence to the behavioural change advice given by the dental team, as well as to check the progress (or not) of further disease.

ii   Look at Figure 7.16 (a). What signs are evident on the radiograph that the LR4 has been resisting the caries process as it has gradually progressed through the tooth?

A: Note the reduced size of the pulp chamber directly adjacent to the lesion. This is tertiary dentine that has been laid down in response to the gradual caries process.

iii   Look at Figure 7.16 (b). What are the classic symptoms of an acute reversible pulpitis? Do you think this distal lesion would be easy to detect on clinical examination?

A: Short, sharp pain of a few seconds' duration, stimulated by hot/cold/sweet stimuli, and poorly localized. Clinically, this lesion may be difficult to detect on visual examination. However, even the wet surface shows a slight opacity on the distal occlusal aspect—drying the tooth would make this more evident. Careful probing proximally may also help to detect the surface roughness of the cavitated lesion. This shows the importance of bitewing radiographs in the examination of such at-risk patients.

iv   Look at Figure 7.16 (c). What is Carisolv™ gel? How does it work? What quality of enamel and dentine has been retained at the base of this cavity and why?

A: Read Section 5.8.5 in Chapter 5 for revision about chemo-mechanical excavation gels. There is caries-affected dentine retained on the cavity base. The enamel margin is sound (it appears slightly frosty as it has been scratched by a gingival margin trimmer hand instrument to help to gauge its strength). If the cavity was to be excavated to sound dentine (yellow and hard) there would be a significant risk of unnecessary pulp exposure, and the restoration margin would end up being very subgingival, thus calling into question the actual restorability of the tooth/the viability of placing a restoration.

v   Look at Figure 7.16 (f). Would you describe the resin composite veneer overlying the Biodentine™ as 'open sandwich' or 'closed sandwich'? What do you think might be the cause of the radiolucent line in the radiograph beneath the Biodentine™ restoration?

A: This is a closed-sandwich restoration, as no Biodentine™ has been left exposed to the oral cavity. Please read Section 2.5.3 in Chapter 2 for the answer to the second part of this question. As Biodentine™ caustically etches the dentine, due to its high pH, it is possible that this radiolucency has been created by this process, and only time will tell (with review radiographs) if this gains mineral and therefore becomes more radio-dense like the surrounding sound dentine.

8

Clinical operative procedures: a step-by-step guide

Chapter contents

8.1 Introduction

This chapter illustrates several minimally invasive operative dentistry procedures used for the successful placement of direct plastic restorations in the posterior and anterior dentition. The procedure list cannot be and is not exhaustive, but has been chosen to give the reader the broadest application of the techniques described. The techniques shown are not exclusive—there are many varied operative techniques for removing caries and placing suitable restorations (see Chapters 5 and 6), but the authors feel that the methods described are simple and achievable for most clinical abilities and in most clinical situations. The experienced skilled clinician is able to adapt the myriad of skills outlined in these examples to best fit the developing clinical situation presented to them.

8.1.1 Cavity/restoration classification

There are several classifications of cavities in the dental literature that attempt to correlate site, size of lesion, and disease activity. The oldest, simplest, and probably most universally accepted is Black's classification (see Table 8.1). This classification was originally used to denote the most common sites for caries to develop, so helping to formulate an idea of the individual's caries risk. Nowadays it is used to describe the site of the cavity or restoration, and is useful for descriptive purposes, communicating between dentists, or annotations in dental records. It must be understood that cavities should not be cut with predetermined geometric shapes according to this classification, but the classification should be used according to the final restoration placed, which will be governed by the biological extent of the caries, the type of material used, and other factors (e.g. amount/strength of tooth structure retained, occlusal factors, etc.).

8.1.2 Restoration procedures

The remainder of this chapter will be dedicated to describing and illustrating the practical stages involved in placing certain types of restoration, outlining in detail the clinical procedures involved (see Tables 8.2, 8.3, 8.4, 8.5, 8.6, 8.7, 8.8, 8.9, 8.10, and 8.11). Discussion of the separate steps will be found throughout the preceding chapters, and these links are highlighted throughout. It is assumed that the clinical need for intervention has been appropriately ascertained and that any necessary local analgesia has been administered prior to commencement of the restorative procedures outlined.

Table 8.1 Black's classification of caries lesions—now often misused by dentists as a purely descriptive analysis of the restoration site

Black's class	Site
I	Posterior restoration contained within the occlusal surface (see also Figure 8.1).
II	Posterior restoration including a proximal surface
III	Anterior restoration including a proximal surface only
IV	Anterior incisal edge restoration
V	Buccal cervical surface restoration

Note that with the increased use of adhesive restoratives, many restorations may involve several of the listed sites and therefore need more specific, accurate descriptions.

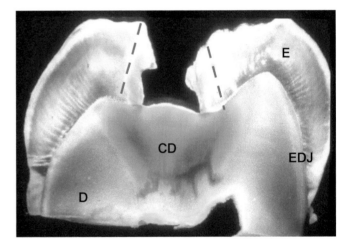

Figure 8.1 A longitudinal section through a cavitated lesion (mICDAS 4), which would also be equivalent to a Black's Class 1 cavity. Note the demineralized, overhanging enamel bordering the cavity, with the undermining spread of the dentine lesion at the EDJ (see Chapter 1 and section 5.9.3 for further discussion of this image). The red dashed lines indicate the extent of enamel removal required in order to achieve a sound enamel margin with supported prism structure, suitable to affect a seal with an adhesive restorative material while still permitting access to the underlying carious dentine. E, enamel; D, dentine; CD, carious dentine; EDJ, enamel–dentine junction.

8.2 Resin-based fissure sealant

Figures 8.2 (a)–(h) illustrate the steps involved in applying fissure sealant. This procedure is also explained in Table 8.2.

Table 8.2 Outline of fissure sealant procedure

Operative procedure	Indication (Chapters 2 and 3)	Preoperative procedures/ isolation (Chapter 5)	Caries removal/cavity preparation (Chapter 5)	Cavity modification (Chapter 5)	Bonding steps (Chapter 7)	Restorative steps	Finishing steps
Fissure sealant (FS) *Composite*	High caries risk, deep fissure patterns, stagnating plaque Newly erupting molars	Rubber dam (Cotton wool rolls/aspiration)	Fissure debridement with prophy paste and rotating brush Sodium bicarbonate air polishing Bioactive glass air abrasion	Wash and dry using 3-1 syringe (10 s)	*Composite:* 37% orthophosphoric acid-etch enamel fissures (20 s), wash and dry (10 s)	*Composite:* FS flowed into fissure pattern, light cure (470 nm) for 20 s	Remove isolation Check margins with probe Check occlusion with articulating paper
GIC/RM-GIC					*GIC/RM-GIC:* 10% polyacrylic acid conditioning of enamel fissures (15 s), wash and dry (10 s)	*GIC/RM-GIC:* applied into fissure pattern, auto-cured/ light cured (470 nm, 20 s)	

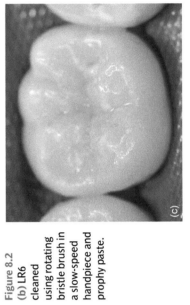

Figure 8.2 (a) Preoperative image of the occlusal surface of LR6 with deep fissures in a high caries risk individual.

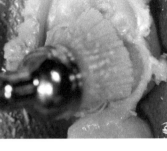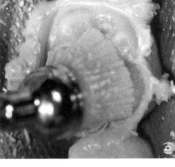

Figure 8.2 (b) LR6 cleaned using rotating bristle brush in a slow-speed handpiece and prophy paste.

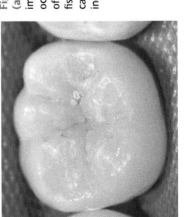

Figure 8.2 (c) LR6 post-cleaning.

Figure 8.2
(e) Etch gel washed off for 10 s and air-dried using the 3-1 air/water syringe. Note the frosty appearance of etched occlusal enamel, indicating creation of micro-porosities which aid the micro-mechanical retention of the resin composite fissure sealant.

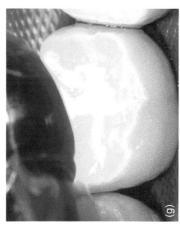

Figure 8.2
(g) Resin composite fissure sealant is light cured (470 nm wavelength light for 20 s) to initiate the addition polymerization reaction of the resin monomers.

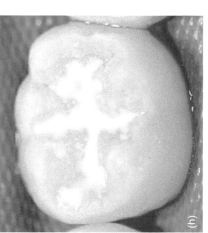

Figure 8.2
(d) 37% orthophosphoric acid etch gel rubbed on to the enamel occlusal surface of LR6 for 20 s.

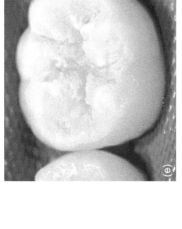

Figure 8.2
(f) Resin composite fissure sealant applied into fissures using a ball-ended dental probe. The sealant flows easily into the fissure pattern.

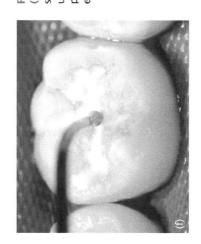

Figure 8.2
(h) Completed occlusal fissure sealant on the LR6.

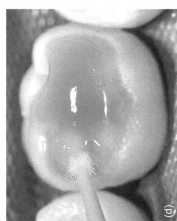

8.3 Preventive Resin Restoration (PRR); type 3 adhesive (selective enamel etch)

Figures 8.3 (a)–(r) illustrate the steps of a preventative resin restoration (PRR) (type 3 DBA, enamel pre-etch). This procedure is also described in Table 8.3 (see also Chapter 7).

Table 8.3 Outline of preventive resin restoration (PRR)

Operative procedure	Indication (Chapters 2 and 3)	Preoperative procedures/ isolation (Chapter 5)	Caries removal/ cavity preparation (Chapter 5)	Cavity modification (Chapter 5)	Bonding steps (Chapter 7)	Restorative steps	Finishing steps
Preventive resin restoration (PRR)	Same as for FS, but evidence of enamel demineralization (mICDAS 1, 2)	Rubber dam (Cotton wool rolls/ aspiration)	Enamel fissure lesion excavated with 330 TC bur, air turbine (Air abrasion—bioactive glass, alumina) Debride remaining fissures with prophy paste/rotating brush	Wash and dry using 3-1 syringe (10 s)	*Resin composite:* 37% orthophosphoric acid-etch enamel fissures (20 s), wash and dry (10 s) *GIC:* 10% polyacrylic acid conditioning of enamel fissures (15 s), wash and dry (10 s)	*Composite:* resin flowed into widened fissure, light cure (470 nm) for 20 s *GIC:* applied into widened fissure, auto-cured/light cured (470 nm. 20 s)	Remove isolation Check margins with probe Check occlusion with articulating paper

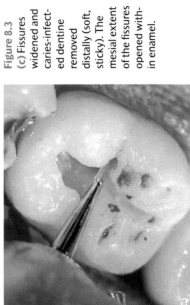

Figure 8.3 (a) Isolated LR7 with deep stained fissures, cavitated and carious in places in a high caries risk individual (mICDAS 3).

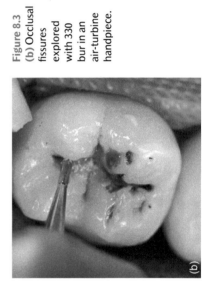

Figure 8.3 (b) Occlusal fissures explored with 330 bur in an air-turbine handpiece.

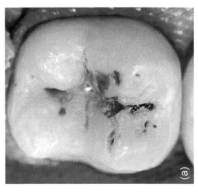

Figure 8.3 (c) Fissures widened and caries-infected dentine removed distally (soft, sticky). The mesial extent of the fissures opened within enamel.

Figure 8.3
(f) LR7 occlusal enamel pre-etched using 37% orthophosphoric acid etch gel for 15 s.

Figure 8.3
(i) Air dried for 5–10 s to evaporate solvent (and thin the layer) until there is no visible 'rippling' of primer on the tooth surface.

Figure 8.3
(l) Flowable resin composite directly introduced into the mesial fissure and light cured.

Figure 8.3
(e) Fine diamond bur is used to remove grossly unsupported enamel and lightly bevel the margins.

Figure 8.3
(h) Type 3 DBA applied (2-step, self-etching primer). Self-etching primer rubbed into all cavity surfaces for 10 s.

Figure 8.3
(k) Type 3 DBA bond/adhesive air-thinned as described for Figure 8.5 (i). Note the shiny cavity floor surface which should be seen before light curing (470 nm, 20 s).

Figure 8.3
(d) Fissure pattern fully opened distally with caries-affected dentine retained at the cavity floor (scratchy but flaky).

Figure 8.3
(g) Gel washed off for 10 s and gently air dried (2–3 s).

Figure 8.3
(j) Type 3 DBA bond/adhesive rubbed on to cavity surfaces.

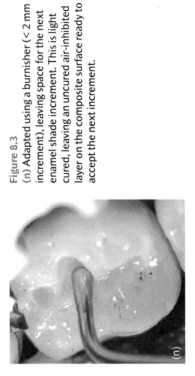

Figure 8.3
(m) Dentine shade resin composite introduced into distal cavity from compule.

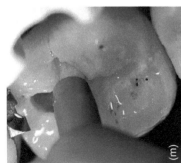

Figure 8.3
(o) Enamel shade resin composite directly introduced into the cavity.

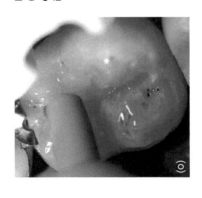

Figure 8.3
(q) The occlusion is checked using articulating paper and finished using polishing points and cups (after removing the rubber dam).

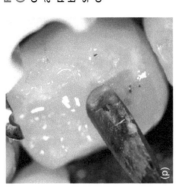

Figure 8.3
(n) Adapted using a burnisher (< 2 mm increment), leaving space for the next enamel shade increment. This is light cured, leaving an uncured air-inhibited layer on the composite surface ready to accept the next increment.

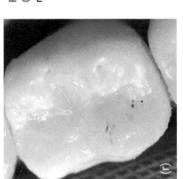

Figure 8.3
(p) Shaped and contoured using a Ward's carver / pear-shaped burnisher and subsequently light cured.

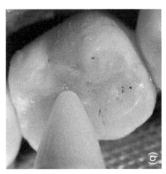

Figure 8.3
(r) The final finished PRR restoration LR7.

8.4 Posterior occlusal resin composite restoration (Class I); type 3 adhesive

Figures 8.4 (a)-(p) demonstrate a posterior occlusal resin composite restoration (Class I), type 3 adhesive. This procedure is also described in Table 8.4.

Table 8.4 Outline of posterior occlusal adhesive restoration

Operative procedure	Indication (Chapters 2 and 3)	Preoperative procedures/isolation (Chapter 5)	Caries removal/ cavity preparation (Chapter 5)	Cavity modification (Chapter 5)	Bonding steps (Chapter 7)	Restorative steps	Finishing steps
Posterior occlusal adhesive restoration: (Class I) All GIC All composite Existing posterior occlusal GIC veneered with composite	High caries risk patient (mICDAS 2); cavitated lesion (mICDAS 3,4) Consider pulp response to sensibility tests Radiographic assessment of pulp proximity	Check occlusion with articulating paper, preoperatively Select tooth-material shade (Vita guides) Place rubber dam	Remove central unsupported/ undermined demineralized enamel with tungsten carbide (TC)/diamond bur, air turbine. Leave sound enamel margin. Peripheral dentine caries excavation (carbon-steel (CS), slow-speed rose-head bur, hand excavator) to affected/sound dentine (lesion depth-dependent). Excavate infected dentine overlying pulp with hand excavator/avoid exposure	Lightly bevel sound enamel margins using fine diamond bur, air turbine Gently round off internal cavity line angles using slow-speed CS rose-head burs Wash and dry cavity (10 s)	*GIC:* 10% polyacrylic acid conditioner rubbed on to cavity walls with micro-brush (15 s), wash and dry (10 s)—removes smear layer and exposes Ca2+ ions for bonding	Mix/dispense GIC into cavity, filling from base upwards (to prevent voids/ improve adaptation to cavity walls). Slightly overfill cavity initially. After 60 s pack GIC into the cavity with burnisher/flat plastics, ensuring adequate condensation. Occlusal morphology adapted with flat plastics and excess material removed while GIC still plastic	*GIC:* wait 3 min for initial set. Check margins/occlusion with articulating paper. Final occlusal adjustments made with diamond burs/stones/sharp scalpel blade. Finish with diamond polishing paste and coat with lightly filled resin for GIC surface protection (dry surface, paint on resin, and light cure (470 nm for 20 s))
					Composite: dependent on which DBA (types 1–4) used (see Table 8.12)	Place *composite* in 2–3 mm increments in stacked angles from base outwards, light curing each increment (20 s). Ensure uncured monomer of the oxygen-inhibited layer on surface of each increment is undisturbed to allow adhesion of next increment. Shape occlusal morphology	*Composites:* Remove rubber dam. Finish surface morphology/ margins with fine diamond burs/discs, check margins/occlusion with articulating paper, polish using diamond grit-impregnated cups/ discs
	Assess occlusal integrity/wear/ marginal failure of > 6-month-old posterior GIC restoration		Remove 2 mm thickness of old, occlusal GIC with diamond/TC bur, air turbine. Leave sound enamel margins				

Figure 8.4
(b) Preoperative view of the occlusal surface of LR7 (mICDAS 2). Rubber dam isolation in place, held anteriorly with medium widget (yellow).

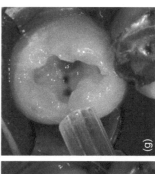

Figure 8.4
(d) 330 bur in air-turbine handpiece used to gain enamel access. Rose-head bur in slow-speed handpiece and excavators used to remove caries-infected dentine.

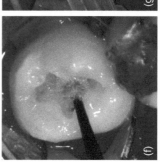

Figure 8.4
(f,g) Adhesive acidic primer rubbed on to cavity surfaces (10 s) using a micro-brush, air-thinned for 5 s and light cured (470 nm, 20 s).

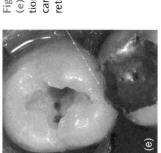

Figure 8.4
(a) Right bitewing radiograph showing multiple early enamel lesions in a high-risk patient.

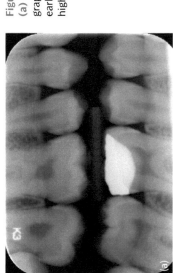

Figure 8.4
(c) Operating view showing rubber dam cut away from nose with paper towel beneath (white). Note that operator's finger rests on lower incisors.

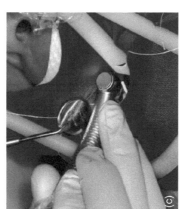

Figure 8.4
(e) Cavity preparation occlusal LR7, with caries-affected dentine retained over pulp.

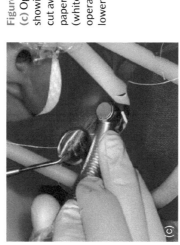

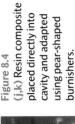

Figure 8.4
(j,k) Resin composite placed directly into cavity and adapted using pear-shaped burnishers.

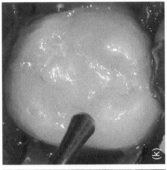

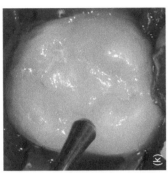

Figure 8.4
(h,i) Adhesive rubbed on to cavity surfaces for 5 s, air-thinned for 10 s, and finally light cured (470 nm, 20 s).

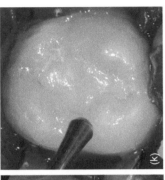

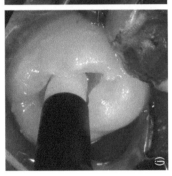

Figure 8.4
(l) Occlusal composite adjusted using fine diamond rugby-ball-shaped bur.

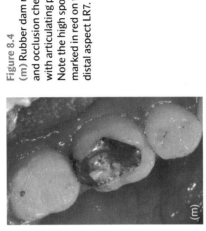

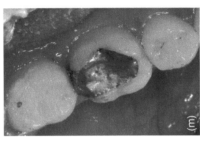

Figure 8.4
(m) Rubber dam removed and occlusion checked with articulating paper. Note the high spot marked in red on the distal aspect LR7.

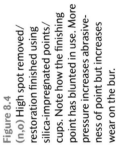

Figure 8.4
(n,o) High spot removed/restoration finished using silica-impregnated points/cups. Note how the finishing point has blunted in use. More pressure increases abrasiveness of point but increases wear on the bur.

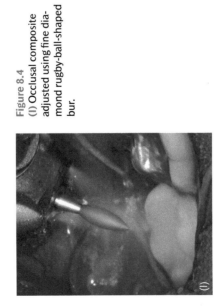

Figure 8.4
(p) Final resin restoration LR7.

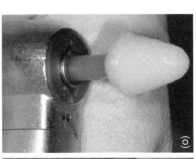

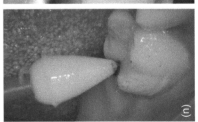

8.5 Posterior proximal resin composite restoration (Class II)

Figures 8.5.1 (a)–(z) and 8.5.2 (a)–(o) illustrate a posterior proximal restoration. This procedure is also described in Table 8.5 (see also Chapter 7).

Table 8.5 Outline of posterior proximal adhesive restoration

Operative procedure	Indication (Chapters 2 and 3)	Preoperative procedures/isolation (Chapter 5)	Caries removal/cavity preparation (Chapter 5)	Cavity modification (Chapter 5)	Bonding steps (Chapter 7)	Restorative steps	Finishing steps
Posterior proximal adhesive restoration (Class II) Contact point present If approximal lesion directly accessible by instruments (e.g. no adjacent contact, rotated tooth), then treat as buccal cervical restoration (see Table 8.6)	Approximal cavitated lesion/mICDAS 3,4. PA radiograph to ascertain depth; pulp response to sensibility tests	Check occlusion with articulating paper preoperatively Select tooth-material shade (Vita guides) Place rubber dam. Pre-wedge adjacent teeth to aid rubber dam placement. Ensure dam can be placed and held firmly cervical to the base of the carious lesion (clamps, wedgets, floss)	Remove unsupported enamel with TC/diamond bur (air turbine), accessing proximal lesion through occlusal surface, just medial to the relevant marginal ridge Once access is gained to proximal infected dentine, remove undermined marginal ridge with excavator or bur. Peripheral dentine caries excavation (CS bur, hand excavator) to affected/sound dentine (lesion depth, moisture control-dependent)—**'box' preparation** Excavate infected dentine overlying pulp with hand excavator/avoid exposure Leave sound enamel periphery, bevelled if possible/avoid gingival papilla trauma	Wash away debris with water from 3-1 syringe and dry (10 s total) Place sectional/circumferential metal matrix band interproximally ensuring tight adaptation cervically with wedges and contact point formation. Circumferential band/retainers may interfere with rubber dam clamps	*Composite:* dependent upon the DBA used (types 1–4; see Table 8.12) *GIC (if difficulty gaining moisture control):* 10% polyacrylic acid conditioner rubbed on to cavity walls with micro-brush (15 s), wash and dry (10 s)	Place *resin composite* in 2–3 mm increments in stacked angles from base of box outwards, adapting against walls and matrix band, light curing each increment (470 nm, 20 s). Ensure uncured monomer of the oxygen-inhibited layer on the surface of each cured increment is uncontaminated, allowing adhesion of next increment. Shape occlusal morphology with carving instruments Mix/dispense *GIC* into box base upwards (prevent voids/improve adaptation to cavity walls). Slightly overfill cavity. After 60 s pack GIC into cavity with burnishers/flat plastics, ensuring adequate condensation. Occlusal morphology adapted with flat plastics	*Composites:* Remove rubber dam. Finish composite surface with fine diamond burs/discs/proximal finishing strips, check margins/occlusion with articulating paper, polish using diamond grit-impregnated cups/discs *GIC:* wait 3–4 min for initial set. Check margins/occlusion with articulating paper. Adjustments made with diamond burs/stones/sharp scalpel blade. Finish with diamond polishing paste and coat with lightly filled resin for GIC surface protection

8.5.1 Posterior proximal restoration - type 3 adhesive (selective enamel etch)

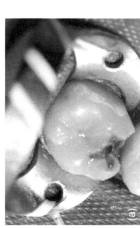

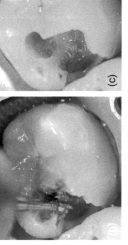

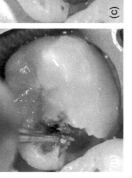

Figure 8.5.1

(a) Cavitated LR8 with mesio-occlusal caries (mICDAS 4) and a lesion present in the distal-occlusal pit (mICDAS 2), both requiring operative intervention. Tooth isolated with rubber dam using a steel wingless molar clamp (threaded with dental floss to enable retrieval in case the clamp dislodges from tooth or fractures).

Figure 8.5.1

(b,c) Using a 330 bur in an air-turbine handpiece, access to dentine caries is improved by removing grossly unsupported and undermined enamel at the cavity margins.

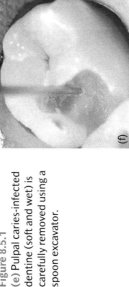

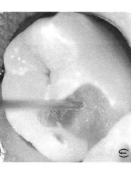

Figure 8.5.1

(d) Size 3 rose-head carbon steel bur in a slow-speed handpiece removing peripheral caries at the EDJ.

Figure 8.5.1

(e) Pulpal caries-infected dentine (soft and wet) is carefully removed using a spoon excavator.

Figure 8.5.1

(f) The cavity floor is scratchy and flaky, indicative of caries-affected dentine over the pulp.

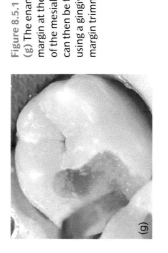

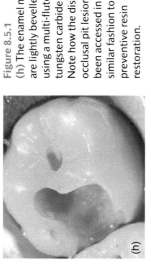

Figure 8.5.1

(g) The enamel margin at the base of the mesial box can then be finished using a gingival margin trimmer.

Figure 8.5.1

(h) The enamel margins are lightly bevelled using a multi-fluted tungsten carbide bur. Note how the distal occlusal pit lesion has been accessed in a similar fashion to the preventive resin restoration.

Figure 8.5.1

(i) Placing the sectional metal matrix band in order to reconstitute the mesial wall of the restoration (see Chapter 5). The precurved, contoured band is worked interproximally.

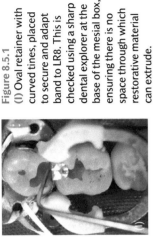

Figure 8.5.1
(l) Oval retainer with curved tines, placed to secure and adapt band to LR8. This is checked using a sharp dental explorer at the base of the mesial box, ensuring there is no space through which restorative material can extrude.

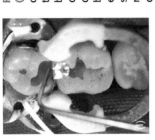

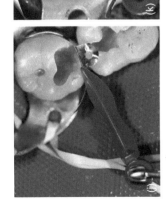

Figure 8.5.1
(j,k) Gingivally contoured plastic wedge is selected and inserted buccally to maintain tight adaptation of band to the mesial surface of LR8.

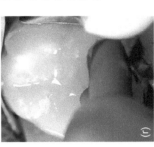

Figure 8.5.1
(o) Air dried for 5 s to evaporate solvent carrier, until there is no 'rippling' of the primer film on the tooth surface.

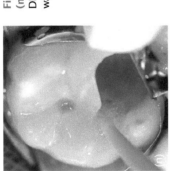

Figure 8.5.1
(n) Self-etching primer (type 3 DBA) is rubbed on to the cavity walls for 10 s.

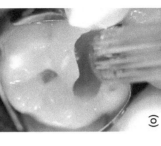

Figure 8.5.1
(m) Enamel margins pre-etched with 37% orthophosphoric acid etch gel for 15 s, washed off for 10 s, and gently air dried for 2–3 s.

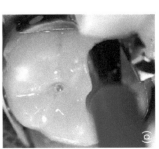

Figure 8.5.1
(r) Occlusal cavity restored with flowable composite. Dentine shade resin composite directly introduced into the mesio-lingual aspect of the cavity LR8.

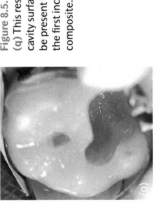

Figure 8.5.1
(q) This results in shiny cavity surfaces which must be present prior to placing the first increment of resin composite.

Figure 8.5.1
(p) Type 3 bond is applied to cavity walls for 10 s, air-thinned using 3-1 air/water syringe, and light cured for 20 s (470 nm).

Figure 8.5.1
(u,v) Final increments are placed, adapted, and light cured, leaving space for the enamel shade composite to be placed.

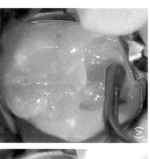
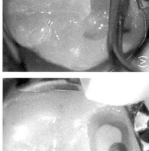

(v)

(u)

Figure 8.5.1
(t) Further 2 mm increments placed and adapted to form the mesial wall of the restoration against firm matrix band and light cured.

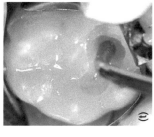

(t)

Figure 8.5.1
(s) Increment is adapted using a pear-shaped burnisher and then light cured for 20 s (470 nm).

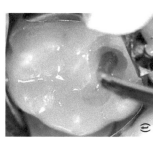

(s)

Figure 8.5.1
(x) Retainer removed with clamp, wedge removed buccally, and sectional matrix teased from interproximal area using special tweezers.

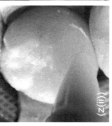

(x(iii))

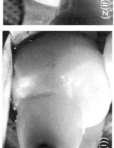

(x(ii))

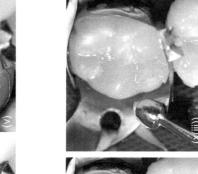

(x(i))

Figure 8.5.1
(w) Using Ward's/Half-Hollenback carver, occlusal morphology introduced in the enamel composite, including mesial marginal ridge, fossae, and fissure pattern.

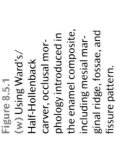

(w)

Figure 8.5.1
(z) Composite surface then finished using silica-impregnated cups and points of reducing coarseness. Diamond polishing pastes can help to achieve a high lustre. Final restoration.

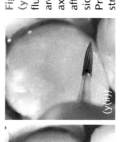

(z(iii))

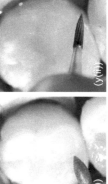

(z(ii))

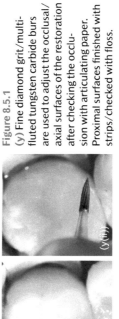

(z(i))

Figure 8.5.1
(y) Fine diamond grit/multi-fluted tungsten carbide burs are used to adjust the occlusal/axial surfaces of the restoration after checking the occlusion with articulating paper. Proximal surfaces finished with strips/checked with floss.

(y(ii))

(y(i))

8.5.2 Posterior proximal restoration - type 2 adhesive, "moist bonding"

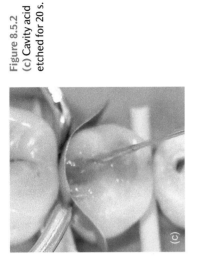

Figure 8.5.2
(a,b) LR5 distal-occlusal cavity (Class II), isolated with rubber dam (wingless clamp LL7 and medium wedget, mesial LL5). Sectional matrix band, wedged gingivally and retained with oval ring.

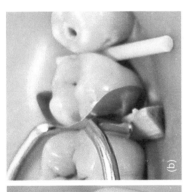

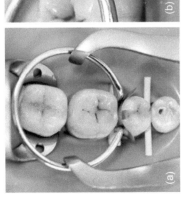

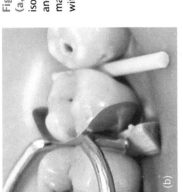

Figure 8.5.2
(c) Cavity acid etched for 20 s.

Figure 8.5.2
(d) Cavity washed for 10 s.

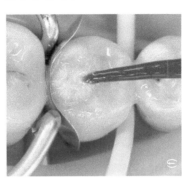

Figure 8.5.2
(e) Cavity blotted dry with cotton wool pledget.

Figure 8.5.2
(f) Type 2 adhesive (primer and bond plus solvent) rubbed on to cavity walls for 5 s.

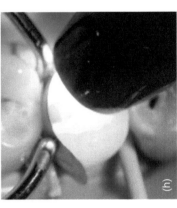

Figure 8.5.2
(g) Type 2 adhesive air-thinned and solvent evaporated for 5 s—look for shiny film on cavity walls.

Figure 8.5.2
(h) Type 2 adhesive light cured (470 nm, 20 s).

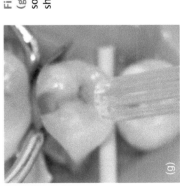

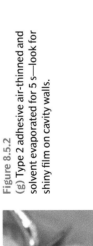

Figure 8.5.2
(i,j) Resin composite placed and adapted into distal box using pear-shaped burnisher. Increments light cured.

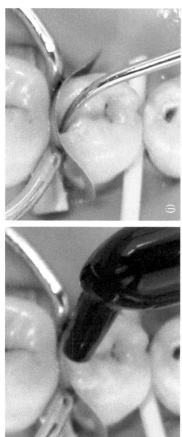

(i)

(j)

Figure 8.5.2
(k,l,m) Resin composite trimmed and finished using fine diamond finishing burs and abrasive polishing discs.

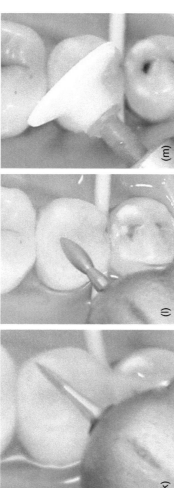

(k)

(l)

(m)

Figure 8.5.2
(n,o) Resin composite finished proximally using abrasive finishing strip, ensuring good distal contour to the final restoration.

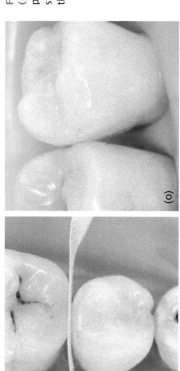

(n)

(o)

8.6 Buccal cervical resin composite restoration (Class V); type 2 adhesive

Figures 8.6 (a)-(n) illustrate a buccal cervical composite restoration. This procedure is also described in Table 8.6.

Table 8.6 Outline of **buccal/lingual** cervical adhesive restoration

Operative procedure	Indication (Chapters 2 and 3)	Preoperative procedures/isolation (Chapter 5)	Caries removal/ cavity preparation (Chapter 5)	Cavity modification (Chapter 5)	Bonding steps (Chapter 7)	Restorative steps	Finishing steps
Buccal/ lingual cervical adhesive restoration (Class V)	Discoloured anterior/ posterior tooth wear (causing plaque stagnation or risk of structural weakness) Cavitated carious lesion/ mICDAS 3,4/ pulp response?	Select tooth-material shade Moisture control: rubber dam isolation often difficult as clamp/dam obscures access to lesion margins Simpler cotton wool isolation/aspiration may be necessary	Caries: remove unsupported and/ or undermined demineralized enamel with TC/diamond bur (air turbine) Leave sound enamel margin (may be difficult cervically). Peripheral dentine caries excavation (CS bur, hand excavator) to affected/ sound dentine (lesion depth dependent). Avoid gingival trauma. Excavate infected dentine overlying pulp with hand excavator/avoid exposure Tooth-wear lesion: ideally air abrade exposed lesion surface, removing stain and surface debris	Lightly bevel sound enamel margins using fine diamond bur, air turbine Wash away debris with water from 3-1 syringe and dry (10 s total)	*Composite:* dependent upon the DBA used (types 1–4; see Table 8.12) GIC *(if difficulty gaining moisture control):* 10% polyacrylic acid conditioner rubbed on to cavity walls with micro-brush (15 s), wash and dry (10 s)	Place *resin composite* in 2–3 mm increments in stacked angles from base of cavity outwards, light curing each increment (470 nm, 20 s). Shape occlusal morphology with flat plastic instruments or cervical matrices, removing excess prior to curing Mix/dispense GIC filling from base up (prevent voids). Slightly overfill cavity. After 60 s adapt GIC with burnishers/ flat plastics to ensure adequate condensation. Surface may be adapted using cervical matrices	*Composites:* Remove rubber dam. Finish composite surface morphology/margins with fine diamond burs/discs, check margins, and polish using diamond grit-impregnated cups/ discs *GIC:* wait 3–4 min for initial set. Final contour adjusted with diamond burs/ stones/sharp scalpel blade. Finish with diamond polishing paste and coat with lightly filled resin for GIC surface protection

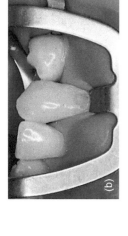

Figure 8.6
(a) Buccal cervical cavity in LL3 with plaque stagnation. Gingival margin finishing on dentine.

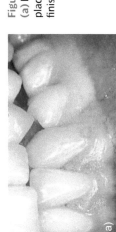

Figure 8.6
(b) LL3 isolated with rubber dam using a Ferrier clamp to ensure good gingival adaptation of the dam.

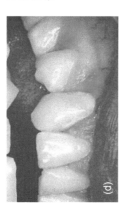

Figure 8.6
(c) Acid etch gel placed on all cavity surfaces for 20 s, washed off (10 s) and air dried for 2–3 s ('moist bonding'—no enamel frosting visible). Adhesive then rubbed on to cavity, air-thinned for 5 s, checked for shiny film, and light cured (470 nm, 20 s).

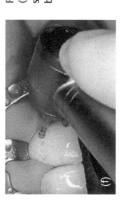

Figure 8.6
(d) Final buccal cervical restoration placed in LL3. Contour achieved using diamond finishing burs and discs.

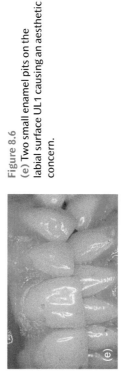

Figure 8.6
(e) Two small enamel pits on the labial surface UL1 causing an aesthetic concern.

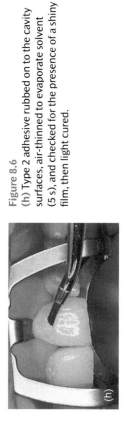

Figure 8.6
(f) Teeth isolated with rubber dam and stain removed with a round diamond bur in the air-turbine handpiece.

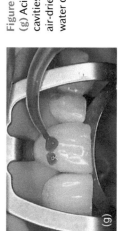

Figure 8.6
(g) Acid etch gel placed on the enamel cavities for 20 s, washed off for 10 s, and air-dried for 2–3 s to remove the surface water droplets ('moist bonding').

Figure 8.6
(h) Type 2 adhesive rubbed on to the cavity surfaces, air-thinned to evaporate solvent (5 s), and checked for the presence of a shiny film, then light cured.

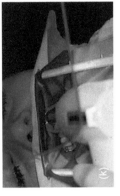

Figure 8.6
(k) Composite light cured. Note the orange filter held in front of the light to protect the nurse's and operator's eyes from the intense 470 nm light.

Figure 8.6
(i,j) Flowable resin composite (shade checked before rubber dam placement) dispensed into cavities and adapted using a titanium nitride-coated non-stick carver.

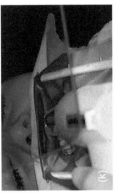

Figure 8.6
(m) UL1 restoration finished using fine abrasive discs.

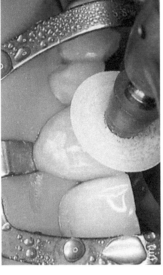

Figure 8.6
(l) Composite adjusted using fine diamond burs with a water spray.

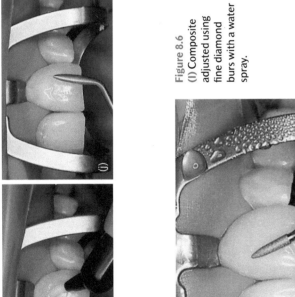

Figure 8.6
(n) Final restoration UL1.

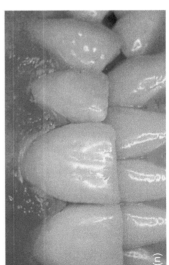

8.7 Anterior proximal resin composite restoration (Class III); type 2 adhesive

Figures 8.7 (a)–(j) illustrate the steps of a Class III anterior restoration (type 2 DBA). This procedure is also described in Table 8.7.

Table 8.7 Outline of an anterior proximal adhesive restoration

Operative procedure	Indication (Chapters 2 and 3)	Preoperative procedures/isolation (Chapter 5)	Caries removal/cavity preparation (Chapter 5)	Cavity modification (Chapter 5)	Bonding steps (Chapter 7)	Restorative steps	Finishing steps
Anterior proximal adhesive restoration (Class III)	Cavitated carious lesion/mICDAS 3,4/pulp response/plaque stagnation Replacement of discoloured/failed restoration	Check palatal guiding occlusion with articulating paper preoperatively Select tooth-material shade (Vita guides—dentine/enamel shades) Place rubber dam. Pre-wedge adjacent teeth to aid rubber dam placement. Ensure dam can be placed and held firmly cervical to the base of the carious lesion (clamps, wedgets, floss)	Caries: remove unsupported/undermined demineralized enamel with TC/diamond bur from palatal aspect (air turbine). Preserve labial enamel wall if possible, to aid aesthetics Leave sound enamel margin (may be difficult cervically). Peripheral dentine caries excavation (CS bur, hand excavator) to affected/sound dentine (lesion depth dependent). Avoid gingival trauma. Excavate infected dentine overlying pulp with hand excavator/avoid exposure	Lightly bevel sound enamel margins using fine diamond bur, air turbine Wash away debris with water from 3-1 syringe and dry (10 s total) Place 15-mm-long clear matrix strip interproximally and wedge cervically (contact point, cervical adaptation of restorative material)	*Composite:* dependent upon the DBA used (types 1–4; see Table 8.12)	Place *composite* in 2–3 mm increments in stacked angles from base of cavity outwards, light curing each increment (470 nm, 20 s) Consider aesthetic layering techniques with dentine and enamel shades Ensure uncured monomer of the oxygen-inhibited layer on the surface of each cured increment is uncontaminated prior to placement of the next, to allow adhesion of next increment Shape palatal morphology with flat plastic instruments, removing excess prior to curing	Remove wedge, clear matrix band, and rubber dam Finish resin composite surface morphology/margins with fine diamond burs/discs/interproximal finishing strips Check margins with probe/protrusive guiding occlusion with articulating paper Polish using diamond grit-impregnated cups/discs

Figure 8.7
(b) The same lesion on UL1; note palatal shadowing.

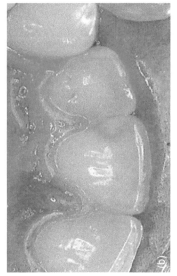

Figure 8.7
(a) Anterior view of a proximal carious lesion (mICDAS 2) on the distal surface of UL1.

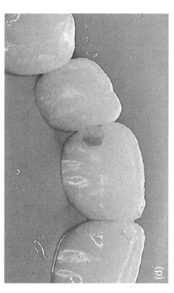

Figure 8.7
(d) The enamel distal marginal ridge cleared through the contact area with the adjacent UL2. Note the brown dentine caries still present.

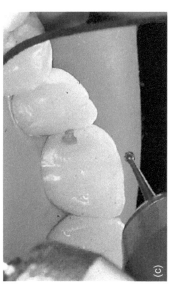

Figure 8.7
(c) Palatal access cut through enamel using a small round bur in the air-turbine handpiece.

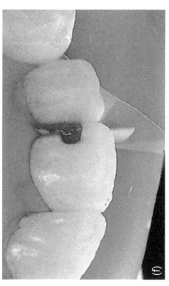

Figure 8.7
(f) Clear plastic strip is placed interproximally and wedged against the tooth surface. The cavity is etched for 20 s using 37% orthophosphoric acid etch.

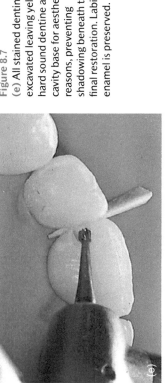

Figure 8.7
(e) All stained dentine excavated leaving yellow hard sound dentine at cavity base for aesthetic reasons, preventing shadowing beneath the final restoration. Labial enamel is preserved.

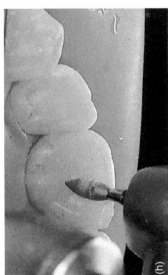

Figure 8.7
(g) Etch is rinsed away (10 s) and dried with cotton pledgets ('moist bond technique') before applying the dentine bonding agent and light curing for 20 s.

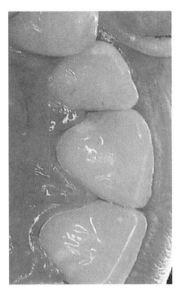

Figure 8.7
(h) Dentine/enamel resin composite placed incrementally and light cured. Palatal surface contour smoothed with rugby-ball-shaped fine diamond composite finishing bur. Occlusion checked with articulating paper

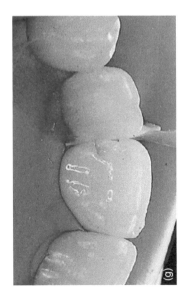

Figure 8.7
(i) Proximal surface finished using abrasive finishing strip (coarse then fine), taking care to preserve the contact point.

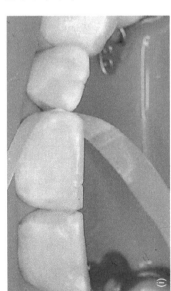

Figure 8.7
(j) Final Class III distal restoration UL1.

8.8 Anterior incisal edge/direct labial resin composite veneer (Class IV); type 3 adhesive (selective enamel etch)

Figures 8.8 (a)-(y) illustrate an anterior incisal edge/labial veneer composite (Class IV) - type 3 DBA (enamel pre-etch) procedure. This procedure is also described in Table 8.8.

Table 8.8 Outline of anterior incisal edge/direct veneer restoration

Operative procedure	Indication (Chapters 2 and 3)	Preoperative procedures/isolation (Chapter 5)	Caries removal/ cavity preparation (Chapter 5)	Cavity modification (Chapter 5)	Bonding steps (Chapter 7)	Restorative steps	Finishing steps
Anterior incisal edge (Class IV) **Direct veneer restoration**	Replacement of discoloured/failed restoration Traumatic fracture of coronal enamel/dentine Aesthetic masking of intrinsic staining, minor alteration of labial morphology Tooth-wear lesions with superimposed caries—high-risk patients	Check palatal/ protrusive guiding occlusion with articulating paper preoperatively Select tooth-material shade (Vita guides— dentine/enamel shades depending on the composite system) Place rubber dam. Pre-wedge adjacent teeth to aid rubber dam placement. Ensure dam can be placed and held firmly cervical to the base of the carious lesion (clamps, wedgets, floss)	Remove old resin composite restoration with diamond/ TC bur, air turbine or bioactive glass/ alumina air abrasion Excavate soft caries-infected and stained caries-affected dentine with excavators/CS rose-head burs Remove extrinsic staining with sodium bicarbonate air polishing, bioactive glass air abrasion. Achieve sound enamel margins at periphery of cavity	Long, undulated bevel cut into sound enamel on labial surface, fine long-tapered diamond bur, air turbine Short bevel placed on the palatal aspect. Sharp line angles rounded off Wash away debris with water from 3-1 syringe and dry (10 s total) Place 15-mm-long clear matrix strip interproximally and wedge cervically	*Composite:* dependent upon the DBA used (types 1-4; see Table 8.12)	Place composite in 2-3 mm increments in stacked angles from palatal aspect of cavity labially, light curing each (470 nm, 20 s) Can use preformed rigid acrylic/ putty matrix outlining the palatal contour, incisal/mesial/ distal margins; interproximal strips cannot be used with matrices Consider aesthetic layering techniques with dentine and enamel shades Ensure uncured monomer of the oxygen-inhibited layer on the surface of each cured increment is uncontaminated, to allow adhesion of next increment Shape morphology with Ward's/Half-Hollenback carver, removing excess	Remove wedge, clear matrix band, and rubber dam. Finish resin composite surface morphology/ margins with fine diamond burs/ discs/interproximal finishing strips Check margins with probe/protrusive guiding occlusion with articulating paper Polish using diamond grit-impregnated cups/ discs

Figure 8.8

(a) UL1 mesio-incisal enamel–dentine fracture (Class IV) causing sensitivity and an aesthetic concern.

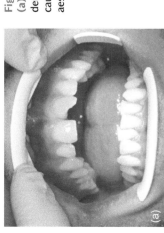

Figure 8.8

(b) Composite shade selected under natural light with hydrated teeth, teeth isolated with rubber dam, and enamel margin prepared with an undulating light bevel on the labial enamel. This is done to prevent a straight-line junction between tooth and final restoration, which would be noticeable clinically.

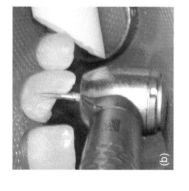

Figure 8.8

(c) Acid-etch gel placed all over enamel margins and labial enamel for 20 s, washed, and dried (10 s).

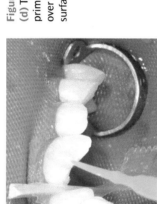

Figure 8.8

(d) Type 3 DBA primer rubbed over the bonding surfaces for 5 s.

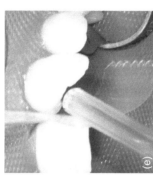

Figure 8.8

(e) Primer air-dried until film no longer ripples (approximately 5 s), removing solvent and air-thinning the film.

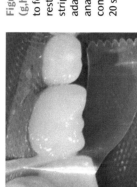

Figure 8.8

(f) Type 3 DBA bond rubbed over the cavity surfaces for 5 s, and air-thinned as before and light cured.

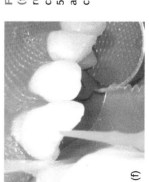

Figure 8.8

(g,h) Dentine shade composite placed to form the palatal wall of the final restoration. Note how the clear matrix strip is wedged cervically for marginal adaptation. The underlying mamelon anatomy is mimicked with the composite. This is light cured (470 nm, 20 s).

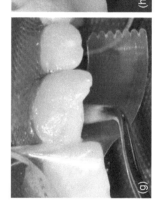

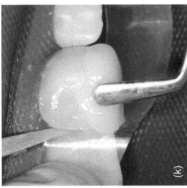

Figure 8.8
(j,k) Roll of enamel shade composite is then teased cervically across the labial surface with the flat plastic, thinning as it blends with the natural tooth along the undulating bevel.

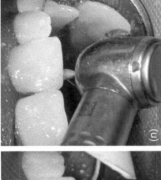

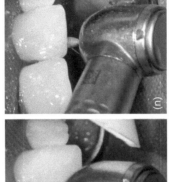

Figure 8.8
(i) Enamel composite is placed as a roll along the incisal edge of UL1 using a flat plastic.

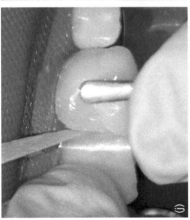

Figure 8.8
(m,n) Margins are trimmed using composite finishing fine diamond burs cervically, proximally, and palatally (rugby-ball-shaped bur).

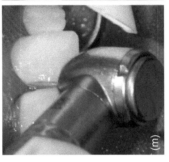

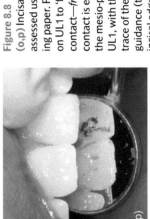

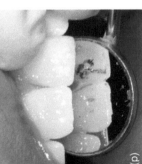

Figure 8.8
(l) This process permits the placement of a smooth layer of composite labially, which is easily finished later.

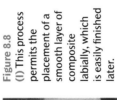

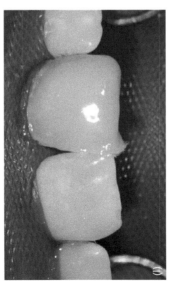
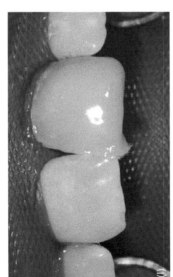

Figure 8.8
(q) This is removed using a fine diamond bur.

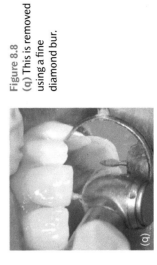

Figure 8.8
(o,p) Incisal occlusion is assessed using articulating paper. Finger placed on UL1 to 'feel' the heavy contact—*fremitus*. A heavy contact is expressed on the mesio-palatal aspect of UL1, with the straight-line trace of the protrusive guidance (towards the incisal edge).

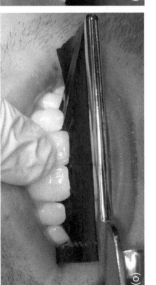

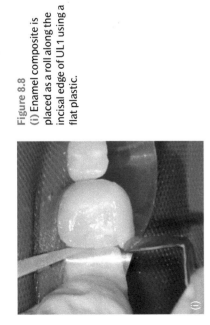

Figure 8.8
(r,s,t) The teeth are dried with cotton wool rolls and the occlusion re-checked this time showing a light contact disto-cervically UL1—normal incisal contact.

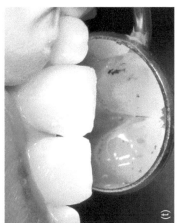

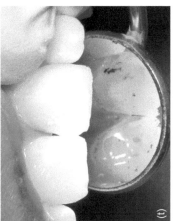

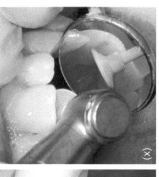

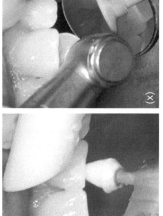

Figure 8.8
(w,x) Composite polished with coarse to fine abrasive points and discs, achieving a final high surface lustre and surface anatomy.

Figure 8.8
(y) Final aesthetic composite restoration UL1 with the patient smiling. Note that the final shade seems slightly darker than the adjacent natural dentition—this is due to dehydration of the natural teeth making them appear whiter. The patient should be warned about this prior to starting the procedure. This will correct itself within a few hours.

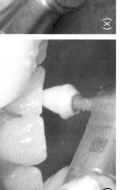

Figure 8.8
(u,v) Proximal coarse/fine finishing strip is worked through the mesial contact, against the restoration subgingivally to remove any excess adhesive, taking care not to remove the contact point.

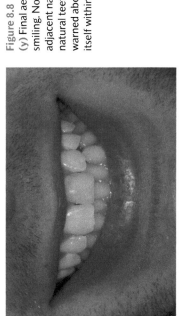

8.9 Large posterior bonded amalgam restoration (courtesy of Dr G Palmer)

Figures 8.9 (a)–(j) illustrate the steps of restoration of a posterior bonded amalgam. This procedure is also described in Table 8.9 (see also Chapter 6).

Table 8.9 Outline of large posterior amalgam restoration

Operative procedure	Indication (Chapters 2 and 3)	Preoperative procedures/isolation (Chapter 5)	Caries removal/ cavity preparation (Chapter 5)	Cavity modification (Chapter 5 and 6)	Bonding steps (Chapter 7)	Restorative steps	Finishing steps
Large posterior amalgam restoration	Heavily broken down coronal tooth structure High load-bearing, large restoration Core build-up for posterior root-filled teeth Difficult moisture control conditions	Check occlusion preoperatively with articulating paper Cotton wool rolls/ aspiration or rubber dam isolation if possible	Cavity/defect already present—access cavity from endodontic treatment, fractured cusps Caries—biologically excavate to sound dentine using hand excavators/CS rose-head burs Remove undermined/ unsupported enamel (diamond/TC burs, air turbine)	Undercut dentine at diametrically opposite aspects of cavity (CS rose-head bur), if remaining tissue permits this Round off sharp internal line angles. Smooth cavity base Indirect pulp capping over blushing pulp with low-viscosity GIC. Wash away debris and dry (10 s) Place circumferential matrix band, wedging the cervical aspect interproximally	*Bonded amalgams*: use auto-/dual-cure resin cement (e.g. Panavia™)	Triturate high-Cu alloy, plug and condense incrementally from the base of the cavity outwards, ensuring adaptation against walls/matrix Slightly overfill cavity and carve back to occlusal level and morphology using carvers (Ward's, Half-Hollenback), flat plastics Work quickly but not hastily!	Remove matrix band. Take care not to fracture/dislodge marginal ridges Check occlusion with articulating paper/ interproximal overhangs with dental floss/finishing abrasive strips Remove high spots with excavator/Mitchell's trimmer or amalgam finishing burs if required Burnish occlusal surface and margins for smooth finish and good adaptation Wipe occlusal surface with slightly damp cotton wool pledget for final surface finish

Figure 8.9

(a) Grossly broken down LL6 prepared for an amalgam restoration. Note the two lingual slots (green arrows) and relative undercuts around the mesio-buccal cusp to aid retention (black arrows), and the disto-buccal heavy shoulder preparation to aid distal support (white arrow).

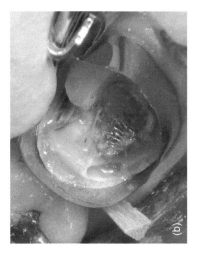

Figure 8.9

(b) Circumferential metal matrix band with retainer placed around tooth and wedged disto-lingually using a wooden wedge to aid adaptation of the distal margin of the final restoration. The band's inner surface is lightly coated with petroleum jelly to facilitate its final removal. To aid retention, a self-etching primer has been rubbed on to the cavity surface and air dried to thin and evaporate the solvent.

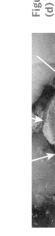

Figure 8.9

(c) A thin chemically cured resin adhesive cement applied using a micro-brush on to the cavity surfaces. This technique is known as a bonded amalgam, assisting retention in very large cavities.

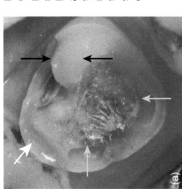

Figure 8.9

(d) The amalgam is condensed into the cavity, filling the volume of the matrix band while keeping in mind the cuspal height of the adjacent teeth. The excess amalgam has been removed around the margins (yellow arrows), thus exposing the edge of the band.

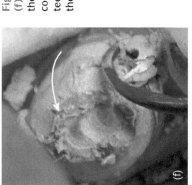

Figure 8.9

(e) After a few minutes, the wedge is removed, and the band is loosened and pushed sideways lingually through the contact area (note the gap, arrowed). The amalgam is supported with a Guy's pattern plugger as the matrix band is eased off.

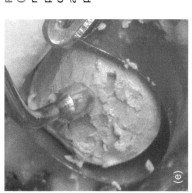

Figure 8.9

(f) Using the curved blade of a sickle scaler, the buccal and lingual walls of the amalgam are contoured, closely following that of the adjacent teeth. The height of the amalgam is reduced to the level of the final cusp tips.

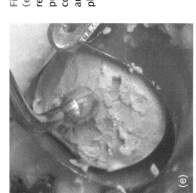

Figure 8.9

(h) Using a Half-Hollenback or Ward's carver, carve in the central fissure pattern (blue line) by joining up the three fossae (green dots). To maintain cusp bulk, try to carve from the fossae up to the transverse ridge (purple lines) and then back down to the adjacent fossa.

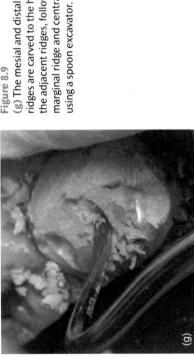

Figure 8.9

(g) The mesial and distal marginal ridges are carved to the height of the adjacent ridges, followed by the marginal ridge and central fossae using a spoon excavator.

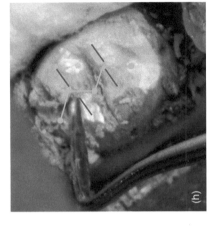

Figure 8.9

(j) After checking the occlusion and margins, the final restoration is burnished and a smooth surface achieved by gently rubbing the surface with a damp cotton wool pledget. (All images courtesy of Dr G. Palmer.)

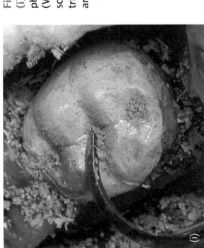

Figure 8.9

(i) Refine the final occlusal morphology and anatomy using carvers (Ward's or Half-Hollenback), sickle scaler, excavator, and/or Mitchell's trimmer, and check occlusion using articulating paper.

8.10 'Nayyar core' restoration

Table 8.10 Outline of 'Nayyar core' restoration

Operative procedure	Indication (Chapters 2 and 3)	Preoperative procedures/isolation (Chapter 5)	Caries removal/cavity preparation (Chapter 5)	Cavity modification (Chapters 5 and 6)	Bonding steps (Chapter 7)	Restorative steps	Finishing steps
'Nayyar core' restoration Amalgam GIC Composite	Posterior root-filled teeth with short, curved root canals Enough cervical coronal dentine must remain to support the final restoration Technique provides retention and strength for the coronal restoration	Rubber dam isolation if possible Cotton wool rolls/aspiration	Use already created endodontic access cavity and natural shape of the pulp chamber Remove coronal 2–4 mm of root-canal filling (e.g. gutta-percha) from the obturated canals, using Gates-Glidden burs	Remove any sharp internal line angles with CS rose-head bur Wash and dry final cavity (10 s) Place suitable matrix as required to replace any missing coronal walls of cavity	*Bonded amalgam:* auto-/dual-cure resin cement G/C: 10% polyacrylic acid conditioner, 15 s (wash and dry, 10 s) *Composite:* DBA, types 1–4 (see Table 8.12) Original Nayyar core described using dental amalgam, but adhesive materials may be used with their own bonding procedures	Triturate, plug, and condense amalgam into the openings created in the coronal aspect of the root canals using narrow Smith plugger/periodontal probe Pack the remaining cavity, slightly overfill and carve back using appropriate carvers For composites/GICs, ensure the root canal spaces are filled without voids, using a dark shade. Place fine capsule tips into canal orifice and back fill (GIC). Light cure composite increments (470 nm, 20 s)	Remove rubber dam/matrix band Check interproximal margins with floss and remove overhangs/finish surfaces with amalgam/composite finishing strips Check occlusion with articulating paper and adjust high spots with carvers/amalgam burs (amalgam), fine diamond burs/discs (GIC/composite) Burnish final amalgam/finish with diamond-impregnated polishing discs (GIC/composite)

8.11 Direct fibre-post/resin composite core restoration

Table 8.11 Outline of a direct fibre-post/composite core restoration

Operative procedure	Indication (Chapters 2 and 3)	Preoperative procedures/ isolation (Chapter 5)	Caries removal/cavity preparation (Chapter 5)	Cavity modification (Chapters 5 and 6)	Bonding steps (Chapter 7)	Restorative steps	Finishing steps
Direct fibre-post/ composite core restoration (see Figure 6.3 in Chapter 6)	Broken down anterior (and posterior) root-filled teeth Relatively straight root canal(s) Technique retains large adhesive coronal restoration and reinforces remaining coronal/radicular tooth structure	PA radiograph of root-filled tooth Choose shade of composite Rubber dam isolation is ideal. Otherwise, cotton wool and suction are essential	Remove gutta-percha root filling using Gates-Glidden burs. Calculate radicular post length from original length of post minus the length of post required coronally. Take into account root canal length, ensuring a minimum of 4 mm gutta-percha is retained apically. Use LCPA Gauge diameter of post from PA radiograph. Prepare post hole using supplied post drills (narrow-wide diameter in stages) Wash and dry post hole (paper points). Holding fibre-reinforced post with college tweezers, try post in for size and fit Section post to required length (if necessary) using a carborundum disc, from coronal end	Round off any sharp line angles on the coronal surface Wash post hole with NaOCl and dry with paper points Clean fibre-post with alcohol and air dry for 5 s	Use self-etching dual-cure resin cement (e.g. RelyX™ Unicem (3MESPE) Activate capsule, automix, attach fine nozzle, and backfill post hole	Insert fibre-post, hold in place, remove excess cement with flat plastic instrument and light cure (470 nm, 40 s) or wait 5 min Apply DBA (types 1–4; see Table 8.2) on to coronal tooth surface and coronal portion of post Place interproximal clear matrix strips to separate adjacent teeth/help to create contact points Incrementally place resin composite, building up dentine/enamel shades if chosen, to provisionalize tooth. Start around post, light cure (470 nm) for 20 s and layer next increment Ensure post is covered with composite	Remove rubber dam/matrix strips Check approximal margins with floss—smooth with composite finishing strips Check occlusion with articulating paper and adjust with fine diamond bur, air turbine/ discs Smooth/polish with diamond-impregnated cups/points/discs

8.12 Types of dental adhesives (dentine bonding agents) – a step-by-step practical guide

Table 8.12 Dentine bonding agents: types, constituents, and practical tips for clinical use.

Type	Smear layer	Etch	Primer	Bond
1 **Three-step** Total etch/ etch and rinse	Remove	37% orthophosphoric acid gel painted on enamel (20 s) and dentine (15 s). Removes smear layer, demineralizes (microporosities in enamel) and exposes dentine collagen fi bres. Wash off (10 s) and air-dry (10 s). May notice frosted enamel.	Contains hydrophilic monomer (e.g. HEMA) acting as bi-functional molecules linking hydrophilic collagen to hydrophobic resin monomers, creating the **hybrid layer**. Exists with a carrier – water. Painted on cavity surface with micro-brush (5 s) and gently air-thinned (2–3 s).	Contains HEMA and other, more hydrophobic monomers. Essentially acts as the unfi lled (or in some cases, lightly fi lled) resin composite. This component is painted onto the primer for 5 s and then light cured (470 nm, 20 s). A shiny cavity surface indicates the presence of the cured DBA, ready for fi rst increment of composite.
2 **Two-step** Total etch/ etch and rinse 'moist bonding'	Remove	37% orthophosphoric acid gel painted on enamel (20 s) and dentine (15 s). Removes smear layer, demineralizes (microporosities in enamel) and exposes dentine collagen fi bres. Wash off (10 s). Air-dry (2–3 s). Blot away surface water droplets (cotton wool pledgets, paper points) – **moist bonding**. If enamel appears frosted then it is likely the dentine surface is too dry and should be rehydrated.	Primer and bond mixed together in same bottle – known as the 'adhesive'. The more hydrophilic monomer (e.g. HEMA) is carried in a volatile solvent (e.g. acetone or alcohol) easing its penetration into the moist dentine collagen fi bres, forming the **hybrid layer**. The combined adhesive is rubbed actively into the cavity surfaces using a micro-brush (5 s). The adhesive is air-dried (5 s) to evaporate the solvent and thin the adhesive layer/prevent pooling within the cavity. Visually check the surface for a 'sheen'; a shiny cavity surface indicates the presence of the adhesive. A dull surface indicates that the adhesive has been blown out of the cavity or has been absorbed into the dentine. If dull, a second layer of adhesive is rubbed in (5 s) and air-dried (5 s) and visually checked. Shiny cavity surfaces can be light cured (470 nm, 20 s) and are then ready for composite.	
3 **Two-step** Weaker self-etching primer	Dissolve	The etch and primer have been combined using acidic monomers, creating a self-etching primer. The acidity of these primers is considerably less than that of acid etch. This acidic primer still contains a solvent requiring evaporation, but no washing is required. The acidic primer is applied with the micro-brush on the cavity walls (5 s) and air-dried (5 s), evaporating the solvent/thinning the pooled primer until no rippling of the applied layer is noticed.		The bond has similar chemistry to unfi lled/lightly fi lled resin composite with some hydrophilic monomers included. This adhesive is applied onto the self-etching primer (5 s), air-thinned for 2–3 s and light cured (470 nm, 20 s). A shiny surface appearance indicates the DBA is in place and ready to accept the fi rst increment of composite.
4 **One-step** Strong self-etching primer	Dissolve	All-in-one systems that present the three stages (etch, prime, and bond) together in one application. Stronger acidic monomers (e.g. glycerophosphoric acid dimethacrylate) etch the tooth surface, dissolving the smear layer, demineralizing and, in dentine, exposing the collagen fi bres to the more hydrophilic monomers to penetrate and form the hybrid layer. DBA premixed and rubbed into the cavity surfaces with a micro-brush (5 s). Air-thinned 2–3 s, visually check for shiny surfaces/no rippling. Light cured (470 nm, 20 s).		

8.13 Checking the final restoration

Once any dental restoration has been placed and finished (of varying size, shape, and material), it is wise for the operator to get into the habit of running through a final clinical checklist before discharging the patient. This involves evaluating the following:

- *occlusion/occlusal morphology/marginal ridge position* (assessed using articulating paper pre- and post-operatively; see Chapter 5)

- *marginal adaptation* (positive or negative ledges, overhangs, excess flash material—assessed using straight probe, Briault probe, or dental floss proximally)
- *tight contact points* (for Class II/III restorations—assessed using dental floss)
- *surface finish* (smooth finish—assessed using a dental probe)
- *aesthetics* (especially in the anterior aesthetic zone, colour/translucency co-assessed by the patient).

8.14 Patient instructions

Depending on the type of restorative material used, the patient should be given appropriate instruction on how to look after/manage the new restoration for the immediate 24- to 48-hour period. In all cases, suitable oral hygiene must be achieved. If local anaesthetic has been used, the patient should be warned to take care when chewing, biting, or consuming hot beverages until the effects have worn off.

- For temporary restorations and amalgam, care must be taken to avoid heavy occlusal loading. Ask the patient to avoid chewing too heavily on the filling for 24 hours.
- For dental resin composites, no further instruction is required. The patient should have been forewarned about the possible shade changes as the adjacent teeth rehydrate over the few hours immediately after the rubber dam has been removed (see Figure 8.7y).

8.15 PubMed keywords

www.ncbi.
nlm.nih.gov/
pubmed/
advanced

QR code image 8.1 Try searching the following keywords on PubMed for relevant further reading. You can access PubMed by scanning the QR code image or at the address .

Keywords

dental restoration failure; dental restoration longevity; restoration repair

9

Long-term management of direct restorations

9.1 Introduction

As has been emphasized throughout this book, minimum intervention oral/dental care involves more than just the minimally invasive operative treatment of the consequences of dental disease. It involves identifying and predicting disease patterns, and concerns the control/prevention of disease by modifying aetiological factors and *reassessing* the adherence to changes in patient behaviours, attitudes, and responsibility. *Monitoring* the oral cavity and restored dentition ensures that the treatment undertaken, and subsequently improved oral health, is *maintained*. This should be accomplished through individualized strategic *recall* regimes. Restorations need to be *reviewed* regularly and occasionally *refurbished*, *resealed*, *repaired*, or *replaced* (see Figures 9.1, 9.2, and 9.3, and Section 9.5). Therefore periodic recall appointments, once an episode of treatment has been completed, are just as important as the treatment itself. It is critical that the patient understands the importance of these recall consultations as part of the ongoing care that is being offered to help to maintain their oral health.

Three aspects of dental care need to be assessed at recall visits:

- the overall state of the patient's oral and dental health (review)
- the individual patient's longer-term response/adherence to previous preventive advice and/or treatment, in moderating any aetiological factors that could cause future dental disease (reassessment)
- the status and quality of the restorations present (monitoring and maintenance).

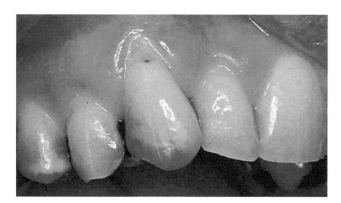

Figure 9.1 Corrosion products from a distal amalgam in the UR3 causing coronal discoloration which the patient complained about—an example of aesthetic restoration failure.

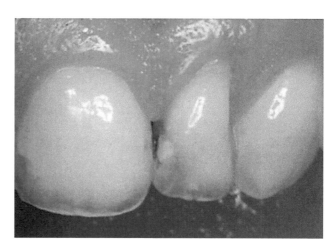

Figure 9.2 An aged, discoloured mesial resin composite restoration on UL2. This caused aesthetic concerns for the patient, who requested its replacement.

Q9.1: What restorative material should be used to replace the amalgam shown in Figure 9.1?

Q9.2: What would be the difficulty faced by the dentist when replacing the Class III restoration shown in Figure 9.2?

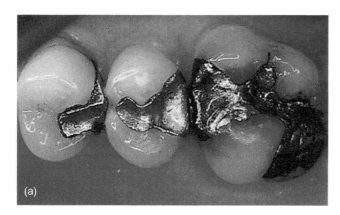
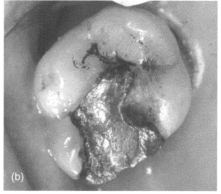

Figure 9.3 (a) A series of old, ditched, and partly corroded amalgam restorations, that were observed on clinical examination to be cleansable and not causing direct problems to the patient. Although the margins and occlusal surfaces are not perfect, should these amalgams be classified as failed restorations? (b) A ditched amalgam UL7 with a marginal defect large enough to accommodate the tip of a periodontal probe, accumulating plaque. A combination of refurbishment with repair or replacement in this case would facilitate plaque control.

9.2 Restoration failure

The potential causes of restoration failure have been identified and outlined in Table 9.1. It is important to appreciate that the causes of restoration and tooth failure (see Table 9.2) are often multifactorial in nature. Indeed, as the causes of both tooth and restoration failure are inextricably linked, it is wise to consider them together, as a *tooth–restoration complex*.

9.2.1 Aetiology

The multifactorial aetiology of restoration failure is often due to manifestations of inherent long-term weaknesses in the mechanical properties of different restorative materials (e.g. poor edge strength, wear,

compressive strength, water absorption, etc.) and/or problems with the technical application of the restorative material for the chosen clinical situation (i.e. incorrect choice of material and poor placement technique).

9.2.2 Choice of restorative material

The chemistry and physical properties of the different direct, plastic restorative dental materials at a dentist's disposal have been discussed in Chapter 7. Restorative material longevity will be affected by:

Table 9.1 Causes of restoration failure and the criteria used to assess this failure, with clinical comments; it is vital to appreciate that multiple aetiologies of restoration failure are common and must be considered alongside the causes of tooth failure—the tooth–restoration complex

Restoration failure criteria	Causes and clinical comments
Colour match (aesthetics)	• Important to get the patient's views, especially in the anterior aesthetic zone—they may or may not be concerned. Ability to manage patient expectations is important at the outset of any treatment offered • Underlying discoloration from stained dentine • Superficial discoloration from marginal/surface staining • Underlying discoloration from corrosion products (e.g. amalgam; see Figure 9.1) • Aged tooth-coloured restorative materials become stained and discoloured due to water/food stain (tannin) absorption leading to a gradual change in optical properties (see Figure 9.2)

Margin integrity	• Loss of margin integrity (*allowing plaque stagnation*) caused by:
	  • long-term creep/corrosion/ditching of amalgams (see Figure 9.3)
	  • margin shrinkage of resin composites/bonding agent (see Figure 9.4)
	  • margin dissolution/shrinkage (on dessication) of glass ionomer cements
	  • margin chipping under occlusal loading due to poor restoration edge strength
	  • presence of ledges/overhangs, poor contour of margins (see Figure 9.5)
	• If the patient can keep the failed margin plaque- and recurrent caries-free and it is not of aesthetic/functional concern, this partial loss of integrity may not be a strong indicator to repair/replace the restoration

Margin discoloration	• Micro-/macro-defects at the tooth–restoration interface will permit exogenous stain (e.g. food stains) to penetrate along the outer perimeter of the restoration as well as towards the pulp • Poor aesthetics (see Figure 9.6) • An indication of margin integrity failure? • Not necessarily an indication of secondary/recurrent caries/caries associated with restorations/sealants (CARS)

Loss of bulk integrity	• Restorations may be bulk fractured/partially or completely lost due to:
	  • heavy occlusal loading—inadequate occlusal assessment before restoring the tooth (see Figure 9.7)
	  • poor cavity design leading to weakened, thin-section restorations (especially for amalgams; see Figure 9.8)
	  • poor bonding technique/contamination leading to an adhesive bond failure and lack of retention
	  • inadequate placement procedures (condensation technique/curing) causing intrinsic material structural weaknesses (e.g. voids, 'soggy bottom' in resin composites)
	• Patients will often complain of a 'hole in the tooth' where food debris is trapped—↑ caries risk (see Figure 9.9)
	• Bulk loss of restoration or occlusal wear may affect the bite/occlusal scheme (see Figures 9.10 and 9.11)

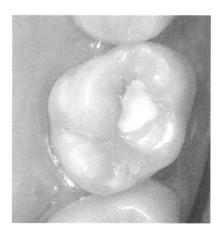

Figure 9.4 Occlusal resin composites on UL6. Note the poor aesthetics and margin staining/breakdown. This restoration would be clinically easier to replace than to repair, due to its small size, in a high caries risk patient with continuing poor oral hygiene, as plaque stagnation will be a concern at the defective restoration margin.

- the differences in physical properties of each material (e.g. bulk amalgam has the greatest strength and resistance to wear, glass ionomer cement (GIC) has limited long-term wear resistance, resin composites exhibit volumetric shrinkage)

- the occlusal loading placed on individual restorations (which might cause some materials to wear/fatigue/fracture more quickly than others)

- the rapid development of dental material science—as the mechanical properties and placement techniques are being refined continuously, so the longevity of new materials will surely improve

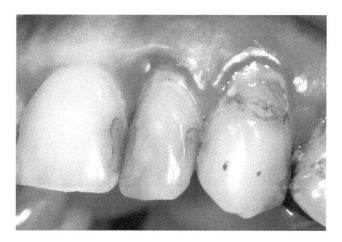

Figure 9.6 Marginal staining evident on the resin composite restorations, distal UL1, mesial and distal UL2, and buccal cervical UL3. The patient complained of poor aesthetics. Note the plaque accumulation at the gingival margins of UL2 and UL3, posing a caries risk in these areas.

Q9.4: Look at Figure 9.6. What periodontal condition has been caused by the accumulated plaque, and what is its relevance when replacing the restorations?

- the simplicity of the clinical handling characteristics of the material (the easier it is to manipulate by the nurse/dentist, and the fewer stages required for its placement, the less opportunity there is for iatrogenic weaknesses to be introduced)

- in addition to the previous point, the clinical skill of the operator. It is these last two points that are most critical in affecting restoration longevity in modern conservative dentistry.

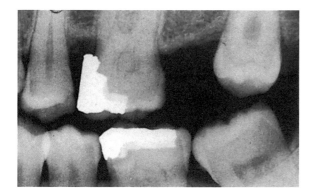

Figure 9.5 A bitewing radiograph of an overhanging (positive ledge) radio-opaque amalgam restoration on the mesial aspect of UL6. Due to plaque stagnation, mesial alveolar bone loss has occurred, along with radiographic evidence of caries (radiolucency beneath the overhang—care is needed to distinguish this from radiographic cervical burnout).

Q9.3: Look at Figure 9.5. What has caused this positive ledge to occur?

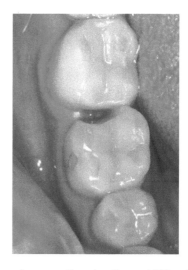

Figure 9.7 The resin composite restoration on LR6 has fractured at the distal marginal ridge due to a heavy occlusal contact with the opposing cusp.

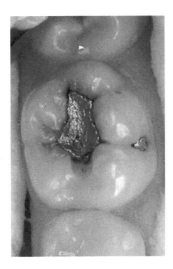

Figure 9.8 A partially fractured occlusal amalgam restoration in LL6.

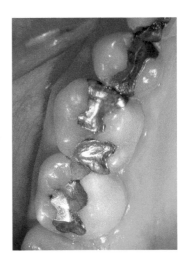

Figure 9.9 Fractured amalgam restorations UR7 mesial and UR4 distal, which need repair due to plaque stagnation and recurrent caries (CARS).

Q9.5: What factors have resulted in the fracture shown in Figure 9.8?

Clinical research studies and statistical meta-analyses of past clinical data have attempted to answer objectively the question of how long restorations should last (see QR code image 9.1). However, due to the numerous uncontrollable variables already mentioned (primarily the operator and the patient), obtaining a precise figure is impossible and arguably irrelevant! Often quoted *average* age ranges of restorations at the time of replacement are as follows:

- amalgam restorations: 10–15 years
- resin composite restorations: 5–8 years
- GIC restorations: 3–5 years.

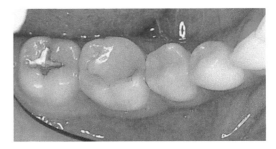

Figure 9.10 Occlusal wear on resin composite restoration LR6.

Q9.6: Look at Figure 9.10. Does this finding necessitate the replacement of this restoration?

QR code 9.1 Scan this code with your mobile device to access MI Compendium, an online resource of collected systematic reviews of MI dentistry techniques and materials.

www.mi-compendium.org

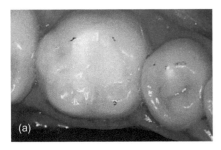

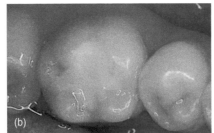

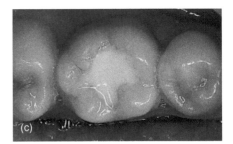

Figure 9.11 (a) Posterior occlusal restoration on LL6 at time of placement (blue marks on teeth are made by articulating paper to check the occlusion). (b) The same restoration 5 years after placement, showing early signs of occlusal wear. (c) The same restoration 9 years after placement, with further loss of occlusal definition. The margins were intact and there were no symptoms from this tooth, but the aesthetics were a little compromised. This does not constitute a restoration failure, and the restoration can continue to be monitored.

However, this does not mean that all GICs, for example, will fail catastrophically after 5 years, or that all amalgams will last for 15 years without any problems. The hotly debated issue regarding the assessment criteria for designating failure (see Section 9.2.3) rears its head when considering the previously cited longevity figures. It must be appreciated that the weighted clinical importance of some of the criteria for failure assessment (outlined in Table 9.1) will be dependent on the restorative material being assessed. For example, when considering aesthetics as an assessment of restoration failure, a black, tarnished amalgam with ditched, corroded margins on a premolar tooth may be considered still functional (as it probably would be detrimental to the remaining tooth structure to replace it), whereas a mildly partially stained resin composite may be considered seriously for repair/replacement (as the repair procedure is perceived to be relatively simple and non-destructive by dentists). Which restoration has actually 'failed'? The most useful answer to the lead question in this section is one given by an experienced operator who has monitored their own patients over many years and has seen failed restorations they were responsible for placing, appreciated the causes of failure, and then repaired/replaced them. This individual can give an honest estimate of the longevity of the restorations placed by their own hand, incorporating into this the individual patient factors.

9.2.3 How may restoration outcome be assessed?

There are several indices available to clinical researchers to help to evaluate the causes and time lines for failure of restorations made from different dental materials (USPHS, Ryge & Snyder, and Hickel criteria to name but three; see QR code image 9.2). However, interpretation of collected, pooled data depends on what is designated a failure in the first instance. A restoration's success may be judged on:

- its clinical or radiographic appearance and technical form
- its clinical function
- whether the tooth is pain-/caries-free.

 QR code 9.2 Scan this code with your mobile device to access the Hickel citeria.

www.ncbi.
nlm.nih.gov/
pubmed/
20847997

When assessing patients in dental practice, either on primary examination or at the recall consultation, the aspects of a restoration to be assessed are shown in Table 9.1. Each of the criteria can be given scores on a numerical scale depending on the degree of 'failure.' Restoration failure is mechanical in origin. However, with experience and consideration of the clinical knowledge of the patient and the patient's views, the clinician is able to make a judgement as to the degree of failure and the necessity of operative intervention, in most cases. Note that a 'failed' restoration may require replacement in one patient, but a similar 'failure' in another patient may be accepted without operative

intervention, depending on other factors. Therefore the decision as to whether to replace/repair the tooth–restoration complex will depend on input from both the experienced dentist and the patient.

9.2.4 How long should restorations last?

There are numerous factors that affect the answer to this important question that many patients will, quite reasonably, ask:

- The caries risk status of the patient (the higher the caries risk for a prolonged period of time, the less likely it is for restorations, independent of the restorative material used, to last as long without problems due to poor patient adherence to preventive regimes/maintenance of oral hygiene).
- The age of the patient. When clinical data from adolescents and adults are compared, it is found that restorations last longer in adults. This may reflect the susceptibility of younger people to caries, or differences in attitude/abilities with regard to dental care.
- The type and size/surface area of restorations. Smaller restorations with a reduced surface area exposed to the oral environment are easier to place and are easier for the patient to clean, as their margins will be more easily accessible to effective oral hygiene procedures and so will last longer than larger ones, if maintained.
- The restorative material used in the correct situation (see Section 9.2.2).
- The diagnostic criteria used by the dentist. This is particularly important with regard to recurrent/secondary caries (CARS), because this is the most common reason dentists give for replacing restorations (see later).
- The age and clinical experience of the operator. Young dentists, with less clinical experience, tend to replace more restorations than older dentists, as they have been exposed less to the deleterious consequences of the destructive operative restorative cycle on the natural life of teeth in their patients.
- Whether the dentist is reviewing their own work or that of another dentist. Changing dentists puts a patient 'at risk' of the diagnosis of failed restorations, and again is dependent on the criteria used to define failure, but this time without any prior background clinical information as to how and why the original restoration was placed.
- The care/attitude/motivation of the patient in maintaining their oral/dental health. Restorations are only ever as good as the operator placing them and the patient looking after them.

The actual answer to the question heading this section is 'It doesn't matter'! In the modern era of minimum intervention dental healthcare and minimally invasive operative treatments advocated throughout this text, the critical question to ask regarding the measure of a successful outcome of dental therapy/treatment is not necessarily about the technical quality and/or status of the restorations placed, but whether natural tooth structure and pulp sensibility have been preserved long term. It is the profession's duty to concern itself, along with the patient, with the maintenance of natural oral/dental health and pulp vitality as opposed to purely that of the restorations/prostheses placed to repair the consequences of dental disease. It is important to remember that none of the man-made materials used to repair/replace natural tooth come close to replicating the qualities of natural tooth structure. These materials will always fail over varying periods of time, and will eventually be replaced by more recently developed products in materials technology, but these will still not be as good as biological tissues themselves. Therefore assessment of successful outcome should no longer be concerned with the simple overall longevity of restorations, but with the level of biological response that they elicit in the tooth and the ease with which they can be repaired when the time comes, without detriment to the remaining viable tooth. Thus this section should perhaps be titled 'How long should restored teeth last?'

9.3 Tooth failure

Teeth can fail for *mechanical/structural* reasons and/or *biological* reasons, either together with, or independently from, restoration failure (the tooth–restoration complex) (see Table 9.2).

Table 9.2 Causes of tooth failure

Tooth failure		Comments
Mechanical	Enamel margin	• Poor cavity design can leave weak, unsupported/undermined enamel margins which fracture under occlusal load
		• Cavity preparation techniques (burs) cause subsurface micro-cracks within the body of the enamel, so undermining the surface (see Chapter 5, Figure 5.34)
		• Adhesive shrinkage stresses on prisms at the enamel surface can cause them to be pulled apart, leading to cohesive marginal failure in the tooth structure, resulting in a micro-leakage risk (see Figure 9.12)
	Dentine margin	• Adhesive bond to hydrophilic dentine results in a poorer-quality bond (compared with that with sound enamel), which hydrolyses over time, leading to increased risk of micro-leakage
		• Deep proximal cavities often have exposed margins on dentine. Poor moisture control leads to compromised bonding technique, in turn increasing the risk of micro-leakage
	Bulk coronal/ cusp fracture	• Large restorations will weaken the coronal strength of the remaining hard tissue
		• Loss of marginal ridges/peripheral enamel will weaken the tooth crown
		• Cusps absorb oblique loading stresses and are prone to leverage/fracture (see Figure 9.13)
		• Can cause symptoms of food-packing, sensitivity
	Root fracture	• Often root-filled, heavily restored teeth (with post-core-crown) under heavy occlusal/lateral loads
		• Traumatic injury
		• Symptoms are variable (pain, mobility, tenderness on biting), but radiographic assessment is not always easy to interpret
Biological	Recurrent/ secondary/ caries/CARS	• New caries at a tooth–restoration gap with plaque biofilm accumulation and stagnation (see Figure 9.14)
		• Detected clinically or with radiographs (can be difficult to interpret)
		• Margin stain is not an indicator of recurrent caries (CARS)
		• Can affect a section of margin and not the whole restoration
	Pulp status	• Heavily restored teeth are more liable to pulp inflammation due to the original disease or the invasive direct operative treatment (see Figure 9.15)
		• Iatrogenic damage or ongoing disease may cause pulp pathology/necrosis
	Periodontal disease	• Examination of the periodontium is required for loss of attachment, pocket depths, and bone levels (see Figure 9.16)
		• Can be exacerbated by poor margin adaptation of restorations (causing plaque and debris stagnation)/margins encroaching into the periodontal biological width

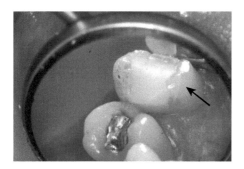

Figure 9.12 A resin composite restoration in a maxillary premolar with a fine enamel crack evident on the palatal cusp (white line) remote to the tooth–restoration interface (arrow).

Q9.7: What has caused the enamel crack shown in Figure 9.12?

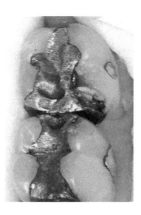

Figure 9.13 The mesiobuccal cusp of LR7 has fractured off due to excessive loading of the weakened crown and possible undermining of the cusp when the cavity was originally prepared.

Q9.8: Look at Figure 9.13. Which coronal structural feature is missing that has contributed to the increased weakness of the remaining tooth structure?

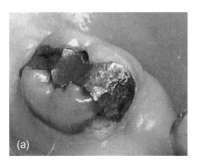 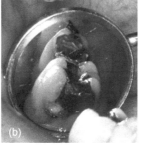

(a) (b)

Figure 9.14 (a) Recurrent caries at the cervical margin gap between the tooth and amalgam in a mandibular molar. (b) Active, cavitated recurrent caries adjacent to an amalgam restoration with plaque retention.

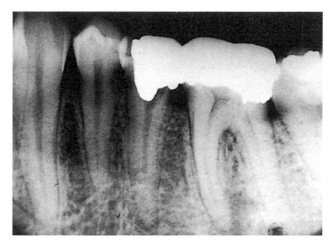

Figure 9.15 Periapical radiograph of a heavily restored LL5; over time the pulp has become non-vital, and there is radiographic evidence of pulpal necrosis.

Q9.9: Look at Figure 9.15.

i   Can you spot the evidence of pulpal necrosis?

ii What anatomical feature might confuse your diagnosis?

iii As the amalgam restoration has not extended into the pulp, why does it appear as though it has?

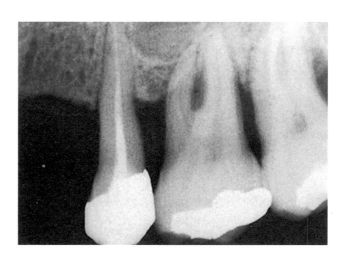

Figure 9.16 A periapical radiograph of a successful coronally restored UL6. Note the loss of alveolar bone support caused by periodontal disease leading to excessive mobility.

9.4 Monitoring the patient/course of the disease

9.4.1 Recall assessment and frequency

The recall visit follows a pattern similar to the initial assessment detailed in Chapter 2. The history will focus on what has happened since the dentist and patient last met. For instance, it is important to recheck the medical history carefully, but questions about the past dental history need not be asked again, except to check that no other dental treatment has been provided in the interim. When the clinical examination is carried out, particular attention is paid to areas noted as important or specifically requiring monitoring (e.g. caries, restorations, tooth wear) (see later).

9.4.2 Points to consider (especially for a previously high caries risk patient)

- Are existing restorations stable?
- Is there any clinical evidence for new lesions/demineralization?
- Is there evidence of lesion progression on radiographs (see Figure 9.17)?

- Are the dietary risk factors still present?
- Is the oral bacterial balance under control?
  - Check oral hygiene (procedures and disclosing solutions).
  - Consider repeating chair-side risk assessment tests (see Chapter 2)
- Has home care (topical remineralizing agents/high fluoride toothpastes, mouthwashes, etc.) helped? Has there been patient adherence to the documented non-operative preventive advice offered?

Visual and radiographic examination may be required, with repeated bitewing radiographs every 6 to 12 months for high risk/caries active individuals (see Figure 9.17). If the patient has modified the causative factors and reduced their risk, becoming caries inactive, then subsequent radiographs may only be required at 18- to 24-month intervals, but these are only approximate guidelines and will be subject to change depending on the patient's response to treatment and preventive advice. The intervals should be judged on an individual patient basis, just like the recall frequency (see Table 9.3).

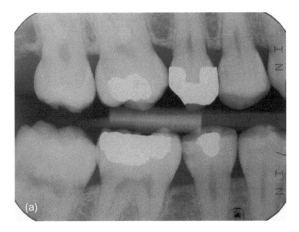 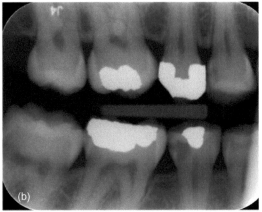

Figure 9.17 (**a**) Right bitewing radiograph of a high caries risk patient with early lesions evident distal UR4 and distal LR5. (**b**) Right bitewing radiograph of the same patient 11 months later showing significant progression of the two lesions. The caries control strategies discussed in Chapter 4 had not been fully implemented by either the dentist or the patient.

Table 9.3 Average recall frequency ranges for patients with respect to lesions present and level of caries susceptibility; note that recall frequencies must be tailored to the individual patient, and the figures presented are purely a guide (for more information about the mICDAS scores, see Table 2.3 in Chapter 2)

Identify	Lesion			No lesion (mICDAS 0)	
	Cavitated (mICDAS 3,4)	Non-cavitated (mICDAS 1,2)			
	High risk	*High risk*	*Low risk*	*High risk (unmodifiable factors)*	*Low risk*
Recall frequency	2–6 months	3–6 months	6–12 months	3–6 months	12–18 months

9.4.3 Monitoring tooth wear

As tooth wear is usually an ongoing problem on first presentation at the dental clinic, it is important to be able to monitor its progress in order to see if it is getting worse, and at what rate, or to see whether the controlling measures advised are having an effect on reducing the rate/stopping further progress. Monitoring methods may include the following:

- *Clinical digital photography*: standardized digital photography of the patient's teeth as shown in figures in this section, with good lighting, can be helpful for comparison over months and years. An overview can be gained from this rather than detailed measurements of any lesion change. Note that, in many countries, full written consent from the patient may be required before images can be captured and stored securely.

- *Tooth-wear indices*: these are clinical scoring systems that are available to permit objective numerical scores of the degree of tooth wear to be noted, reassessed, and compared at a later date. Some indices will also help with the care planning regimen required for the individual patient. Unfortunately, as with many of these indices, they are often complicated and time-consuming to use in a busy dental practice. Their use in research and epidemiological studies is recommended, but in general dental practice their use may be limited. However, practitioner-friendly tooth-wear screening indices do exist that help to give an overview of the patient's existing problem—for example, the Basic Erosive Wear Examination (BEWE) (see Table 2.4 in Chapter 2).

- *Serial, dated study models* (see Figure 9.18): Casts of the dentition can be made from impressions at 12- to 18-month intervals in patients where the tooth wear appears to be progressing, in order to be able to compare the changes and develop future care plans. Again, as with clinical photography, the changes will have to be quite extensive to be noticed. The patient should be given the dated casts to keep safely ensconced in bubble wrap and bring to future appointments. This may also help to evaluate better the attitude/motivation of the individual patient with regard to their tooth-wear problem. Remember that unless the patient appreciates their own responsibility for managing their condition, no form of treatment will be successful in the medium to long term.

- *Profilometry*: Using laboratory-based laser scanners, serial models can be scanned to give accurate changes in lesion dimensions over

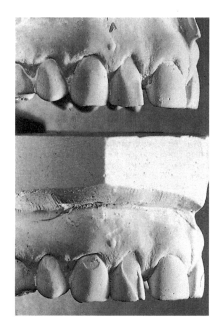

Figure 9.18 Serial study models taken with a 3-year interval showing the progress of tooth-wear lesions on the buccal aspects of UR234.

a period of time. This is a useful research tool at present. Intra-oral chair-side scanners, initially developed for fixed prosthodontic dental applications, are now being developed to measure this detailed level of tooth surface morphological change over time, and may prove useful in a dental practice setting.

As with all cases where the progression of a relatively slowly developing lesion, disease, or condition is being measured, the relative impact of the perceived change on the patient's lifestyle plays a significant role in motivating the patient to alter their behaviour so as to prevent the occurrence of further disease. A patient is less likely to be concerned about a condition that is only developing slowly with little or no detrimental impact on their way of life. However, a rapid obvious deterioration in their health will have more impact, spurring them on to change their lifestyle. The screening index that has the most impact on the patient will require the appropriate level of explanation from members of the oral healthcare team in the clinic. Indices cannot be relied upon without this critical back-up.

9.5 Managing the failing tooth–restoration complex: the '5 Rs'

As was stated at the beginning of this chapter, the long-term maintenance and survival of the tooth–restoration complex are dependent upon regular and careful recall consultations to review not only the status of existing restorations, but also the patient's attitude to maintaining them with the appropriate level of well-executed preventive home care. Nevertheless, all tooth–restoration complexes have a finite lifespan, as has been discussed earlier. Modern restorations can be *refurbished*, *repaired*, and/or *replaced* when deemed necessary by the operator and the patient. The decision to repair or replace a restoration is one that has to be made specifically for a particular situation in a particular patient.

When significant portions of the restoration (> 50%) have failed or the surrounding tooth structure is structurally and/or functionally compromised, partial or complete replacement of the restoration will be indicated. In most other cases, especially where the original restoration material type is known, careful minimally invasive repair of the deficient, fractured, or weakened sections may be appropriate. When removing old adhesive restorations completely, there is a significant chance of enlarging the cavity with a rotary instrument due to similarities in colour of the restoration and the surrounding tooth structure. Therefore other operative technologies may be useful, such as air abrasion (see Chapter

5, Section 5.8.4). Repairing failing portions of an existing restoration is the more conservative and minimally invasive option.

The minimally invasive non-operative/operative management options for the tooth–restoration complex that has been diagnosed as failing may be divided into five categories:

1. *Review* (see Figure 9.11): If only minor defects are evident, such as surface roughness/irregularities without concomitant plaque biofilm stagnation, the restoration can be monitored non-operatively. The primary factor in deciding to review is that by commencing operative treatment there will be no net clinical advantage gained by the patient. It is imperative that the patient is informed of the decision, with an explanation of its rationale, and that this is documented clearly in the notes, for both clinical and dento-legal purposes. Assessment of the patient's caries risk and their responsible adherence to non-operative preventive regimes is imperative. The use of intra-oral clinical photography is recommended to aid the reviewing of restorations long term. Care should be taken to try to standardize the perspective and lighting conditions between images taken. Suitable recall periodicity is required, and this will be dependent upon the attitude and interest that the patient has with regard to their own oral health.

2. *Refurbishment* (see Figure 9.19): This is indicated if there are small defects in the restoration which require intervention, including reshaping, removal of excess material, and/or polishing. If plaque stagnation occurs in such surface defects, and the patient cannot remove it easily with oral hygiene procedures, or there is an aesthetic benefit to the finished restoration, refurbishment is indicated. Micro-abrasion techniques to refresh resin composite surfaces, especially in the anterior aesthetic zone, would be included in this category.

3. *Resealing* (Figure 9.20): This is defined as the application of sealant into a non-carious, defective margin gap and/or surface. This is achieved through the use of flowable resin-based adhesive systems. Sealing a restoration minimally invasively prevents further ingress of plaque and the potential of caries developing.

4. *Repair*: This is the addition of a restorative material to an existing restoration. It may involve operative removal of the defective part of the restoration or modification of the existing retained portion to facilitate retention. A minimally invasive approach aims to restore the failing restoration while preserving the maximum quantity of tooth structure and maintaining pulp viability.

5. *Replacement*: This is the complete removal of the existing restoration and necessary tooth structure to prevent disease progression or to aid retention/stability. It is indicated if there are multiple or severe problems associated with the existing failed tooth–restoration complex, where a segmental repair is not feasible.

It must be appreciated that, in the majority of clinical cases, these categories of treatment are not mutually exclusive and cannot be considered separately. A more extensive surface refurbishment of a restoration together with resealing of its defective margins could be considered as a tooth–restoration complex repair. The categories have been defined to allow a better understanding of the minimally invasive approach to biological tooth preservation. The application of these procedures should not be considered a 'failure' of care, but rather part of the long-term management process of dental restorations. The '5 Rs' MI management protocol will be applied to different restorative materials in the following sections.

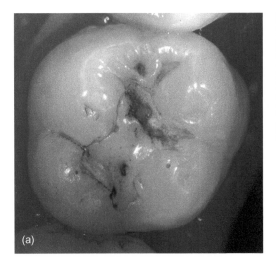
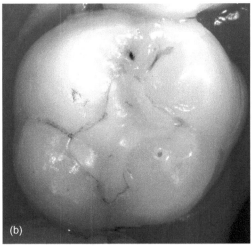

Figure 9.19 **(a)** A maxillary left molar with an old, stained, roughened occlusal resin composite Class I restoration. Especially in an at-risk patient with poorer oral hygiene, this restoration would encourage plaque stagnation. Many dentists would consider replacing a restoration with this appearance. **(b)** The same restoration after it has been refurbished simply using abrasive polishing discs/burs, taking only a few minutes. Its appearance has improved along with its morphology and smooth surface finish. This minimally invasive approach has indirectly increased the longevity of this restoration, as few dentists would now choose to replace it! (Courtesy of L Mackenzie.)

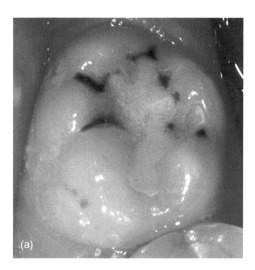 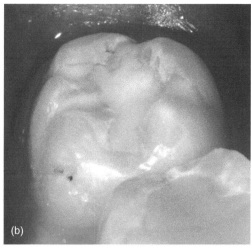

Figure 9.20 (a) Non-carious, stained, and defective margins associated with an occlusal resin composite restoration on a mandibular right second molar. **(b)** The defective margins were cleaned using air abrasion with 27-μm alumina particles, acid-etched for 20 seconds, wash and dried, adhesive placed, and resealed with a resin-based fissure sealant and photo-cured. (Courtesy of Dental Update.)

9.5.1 Dental amalgam

The most common causes of failure of dental amalgam restorations are secondary caries (pathological) and restoration/tooth fracture (mechanical) (see Tables 9.1 and 9.2).

- *Review.* If only minor deficiencies are present in the restoration, such as a minimal surface defect, reviewing the restoration periodically as per standard recall guidelines is a sensible management option. If there is no clinical advantage to treating the restoration operatively, it should be reviewed. Indeed, operative intervention of old, established amalgams can lead to significant levels of tooth tissue destruction, as the corroded alloy offers some 'support' to weakened tooth structure over time. Removing this can accelerate cusp /wall failure, thus complicating the replacement restoration significantly (see Figure 9.3a). Appropriate documentation and informed consent should be obtained from the patient.

- *Refurbishment or re-finishing* existing amalgam restorations (using brown and green amalgam abrasive rubber polishing points in a slow-speed handpiece; see Figure 5.31 in Chapter 5) is a useful treatment for anatomical form defects and for refreshing an old tarnished restoration. The refurbishment of anatomical form and surface roughness involves conservative and simple procedures which can enhance the appearance of amalgam restorations and, indirectly, their longevity, as they are less likely to be replaced by the dentist in the future.

- *Resealing.* The application of a resin composite sealant into a non-carious gap/defect at the margin of an amalgam restoration has been shown to increase the clinical longevity of the amalgam restoration (see Figure 9.21). Prior to application of a flowable resin composite, the amalgam surface and adjacent tooth can be modified using a variety of techniques. Air abrasion, etching with orthophosphoric acid,

and application of a dentine bonding agent are all effective protocols cited in the literature.

- *Repair.* It is relatively easy to remove the remaining amalgam restoration/loose fragment. A tungsten carbide (TC) Beaver bur (see Figures 5.29 (a) and 5.33 (d) in Chapter 5) is used to cut through the amalgam from its centre towards the periphery of the portion to be removed (avoiding contact with the cavity margins). Large fragments are usually dislodged or can be flicked away using hand excavators (see Chapter 5).

  - Cavity margins may be 'freshened up' using rotary instrumentation to remove stain or early demineralized hard tissues, especially if the restoration is to be repaired/replaced using a tooth-coloured adhesive restorative material.

  - Retention has to be gained macro-mechanically via cavity undercuts, slots, or grooves. If replacing the complete restoration, these retentive features will often already feature in the existing cavity design and may only need slight modification. When repairing the damaged portion of the restoration/tooth only, these retentive design features should be cut into the retained portion of the original amalgam restoration to avoid further loss and weakening of the surrounding tooth structure (see Figure 9.22a).

  - Some may advocate the use of chemical retention, using a bonded amalgam technique, in an attempt to conserve the remaining tooth structure, but there is limited evidence for the long-term success rates of this repair technique (see Chapter 7, Section 7.5.3, and Chapter 8, Section 8.9).

  - If the previous steps can be carried out, the repair can be completed using amalgam (see Figure 9.22b). If not, resin composite (including the use of an etch-and-rinse adhesive, types 1 and 2) or chemically adhesive GIC in situations with poor moisture control might be the materials of choice. The margins must be contoured appropriately, avoiding ledges, overhangs, and voids.

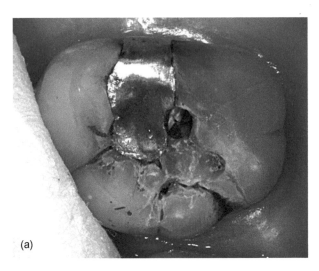

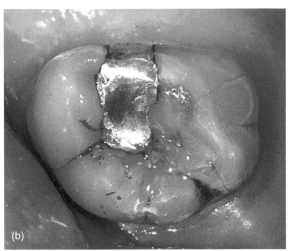

(a)

(b)

Figure 9.21 (a) The occlusal surface of a UR7 with a Class II mesio-occlusal (MO) amalgam restoration. Note the non-carious defect associated with the palatal margin of the amalgam. **(b)** The defect has been cleaned, acid-etched, adhesive applied, and resealed using flowable resin composite. (Courtesy of L. Mackenzie.)

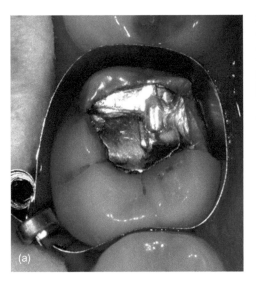

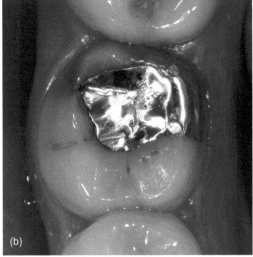

(a)

(b)

Figure 9.22 (a) LR6 with an old occlusal amalgam and a recently fractured disto-lingual cusp. A retentive lock has been cut into what was originally an occlusal amalgam to improve retention for the repair. **(b)** The repair of the tooth–restoration complex has been successful using amalgam. The image was taken 2 years after the repair was originally carried out. (Courtesy of Dental Update.)

> **Q9.10:** Look at Figure 9.22 (a). How else can the amalgam repair bond to the old restoration be enhanced?

9.5.2 Resin composites/GIC

In contrast to dental amalgam, resin composite restorations present a more complicated chemical substrate for repair. There is variation in the chemical composition of resin composites with regard to the type of resin matrix, with additional disparities in inorganic filler quantity and type. The age of the restoration also has a significant deleterious effect on the bond strength between new and old resin composite repairs. Newly placed resin composites, placed incrementally, have cohesion between increments due to the presence of uncured resin monomer after photo-curing—the oxygen-inhibited layer. This degrades rapidly in clinical service and reduces the success of bonding further additions of resin composite for intra-oral repairs.

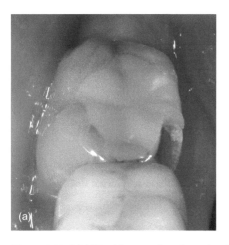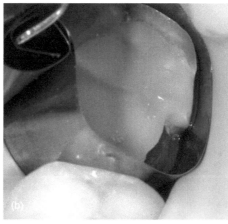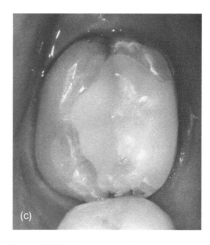

Figure 9.23 (a) LR7 with an occluso-lingual resin composite restoration and a fractured mesio-lingual cusp. **(b)** The isolated cavity walls can be freshened with rotary instruments or air abrasion. The cavity is then silanated to improve the resin composite–composite bond, and adhesive applied and photo-cured. **(c)** The immediate post-operative image of the resin composite–composite repair. (Courtesy of Dental Update.)

Q9.11: What type of matrix system has been used in the restoration shown in Figure 9.23 (b)?

Dentists have been shown to be more likely to intervene operatively with a resin composite restoration than with an amalgam restoration. It has been speculated that this difference may be due to the perceived increased longevity of amalgam restorations in general, and the lack of correlation between margin breakdown and the presence of caries.

- It is more usual to refurbish, reseal, or repair adhesive restorations, rather than replace them completely. Polishing, improvement in surface roughness, and anatomical form of Class I and II resin composite restorations have been shown to maintain an improvement for 3 years post intervention (see Figure 9.19). If there is a gross aesthetic or biological concern, old restorations may be veneered/re-surfaced with new material (the old restoration being resurfaced with an up-to-date, shade-matched equivalent, rather than replaced completely).

- Repair. Use rotary instrumentation to remove the defective portion of restoration. Care must be taken to avoid cavity over-preparation, as it can be difficult to distinguish between the adhesive restoration and the cavity margin due to colour similarities. Air-abrasive techniques using alumina or bioactive glass powders might facilitate this process, due to their inherent selectivity for resin composites and/or grossly demineralized enamel.

- Fresh cavity margins should expose a roughened enamel and/or dentine surface for better micro-mechanical/chemical adhesion.

- *GIC repair*: condition all surfaces with 10% polyacrylic acid for 10 seconds, wash thoroughly, blot dry, and apply/pack GIC (with matrixing as appropriate).

- *Resin composite repair* (see Figure 9.23): acid-etch with 37% ortho-phosphoric acid for 20 seconds (enamel) and 10–15 seconds (dentine), wash thoroughly (10 seconds), and dry.

- Silanating agent may be used to couple new methacrylate-based resin composite to old (painted on the bonding surface of the old restoration and evaporated). This step may be omitted, as it can interfere with the adhesive chemistry of the specific dental adhesive used, and also it may be clinically difficult to separate these two procedures.

  Dentine bonding agent is agitated on to cavity surfaces, gently dried (until no rippling is noticed, indicating solvent evaporation), and light-cured.

  Resin composite is added in small increments, photo-cured, and finished appropriately (see Figure 5.32 in Chapter 5).

- Another factor in the success of resin composite repairs is appreciating the chemistry of the original material and the ability to match new material with old. The use of a dental adhesive also significantly improves outcomes, mainly by increasing the 'wetting' or adaptation of the repairing material.

 9.6 Answers to self-test questions

Q9.1: What restorative material should be used to replace the amalgam shown in Figure 9.1?

A: Dental resin composite.

Q9.2: What would be the difficulty faced by the dentist when replacing the Class III restoration shown in Figure 9.2?

A: Aesthetics—matching the natural translucency from the incisal edge through to the mesial aspect of the UL2. An aesthetic layered composite restoration would have to be placed carefully mimicking the underlying dentine and overlying enamel shades.

Q9.3: Look at Figure 9.5. What has caused this positive ledge to occur?

A: A poorly adapted/wedged matrix band at the cervical margin of the approximal Class II cavity.

Q9.4: Look at Figure 9.6. What periodontal condition has been caused by the accumulated plaque, and what is its relevance when replacing the restorations?

A: Chronic marginal gingivitis. This would need to be remedied with improved oral hygiene techniques prior to any restoration being placed, in order to ensure optimal moisture control during placement of the new composite restorations.

Q9.5: What factors have resulted in the fracture shown in Figure 9.8?

A: Poor cavity design—the mesial portion of the cavity was too shallow and the amalgam fractured under occlusal load due to its inherent weakness in thin section and lack of macro-mechanical retentive features. Inappropriate choice of material—a resin composite might have been a better choice, thereby preventing any unnecessary extension of the cavity.

Q9.6: Look at Figure 9.10. Does this finding necessitate the replacement of this restoration?

A: No. The restoration is fully functional and is not causing any clinical problems.

Q9.7: What has caused the enamel crack shown in Figure 9.12?

A: It has been caused by shrinkage stress from the composite pulling on the prismatic enamel structure and causing cohesive failure in the enamel.

Q9.8: Look at Figure 9.13. Which coronal structural feature is missing that has contributed to the increased weakness of the remaining tooth structure?

A: A missing mesial marginal ridge.

Q9.9: Look at Figure 9.15.

i Can you spot the evidence of pulpal necrosis?

A: Widening of the periodontal ligament space at the root apex, with loss of lamina dura in this area of the LL5.

ii What anatomical feature might confuse your diagnosis?

A: An overlying mental foramen.

iii As the amalgam restoration has not extended into the pulp, why does it appear as though it has?

A: There is an additional buccal cervical amalgam restoration, the radiographic opacity of which has superimposed itself over the pulp chamber radiolucency.

Q9.10: Look at Figure 9.22 (a). How else can the amalgam repair bond to the old restoration be enhanced?

A: By using air abrasion/burs to roughen the surfaces, and then using a resin cement in a bonded amalgam technique. However, there is inconclusive evidence as to whether this actually strengthens the adhesive bond between the two amalgams.

Q9.11: What type of matrix system has been used in the restoration shown in Figure 9.23 (b)?

A: A circumferential metal matrix band. This is required because a sectional band would not extend to help to contour the mesio-lingual aspect of the restoration.

Index